'Finally a book that is practical to do. .

Dr Fabrizio Mancini, Healt
Best-Selling Author of *The Power of Self-Healing*

C000241525

ONE BODY ONE LIFE

DON'T SCREW IT UP!

ANDREW C E GREEN

One Body One Life

First published in 2018 by

Panoma Press Ltd
48 St Vincent Drive, St Albans, Herts, AL1 5SJ, UK
info@panomapress.com
www.panomapress.com

Book layout by Neil Coe.

Printed on acid-free paper from managed forests.

ISBN 978-1-784521-34-9

Dedication

This book is for my Dad. I wish we had had more time to talk. There was so much I did not ask.

Acknowledgements

I wish to thank the following people for their ongoing support, advice and love while I was writing the book:

My wife, Laura, for her constant love, support, patience, belief and encouragement. Thank you Sweet Pea… Love you more!

My three sons, Harrison, Kaspar and Ozzy, whose presence (whilst often disruptive) altered my entire perspective on life.

My Mum, Carol, who has always supported my crazy plans!

The Reflex Spinal Health team. You guys are awesome and provide superb care and clinical excellence. Thank you for all you do.

Steve and Jo, for twisting my arm to sit down and write it, and Mindy for giving me the tools.

Contents

Introduction

Who am I?

"Last 30 seconds, come on lads, push it on," my rowing coach, Bill Mason, shouted through the megaphone. Lungs burning, legs and back going numb, I pushed my body on while feeling the carbon racing shell of the Imperial College Eight scything through the water beneath me. Despite feeling exhausted I always felt amazing, almost euphoric, racing at full speed along the Thames and up to the Putney Embankment. It must have been the penultimate stroke of that particular training row when I felt a sudden, intense spasm of sharp pain jolting through the base of my spine and into the right side of my lower back. Fortunately, we ended that timed piece and the whole crew ground to a halt, bending over their oars as they sucked in precious oxygen. I remember to this day bracing my hands on the sides of the boat and lifting myself off the seat to take the load off my back and the pain that was now starting to throb intensely.

By the time we had rowed the eight, very slowly, back to the shore my back was stiffening up so fast it was tough to get out of the boat. The worst thing was that this was approximately six weeks from the 1992 Under-23 World Rowing Championships (then called the Nations Cup) and I had been selected to row for Great Britain. I was 21 years old, and this was probably the single most important thing that had ever happened to me in my life. It was certainly one of the achievements that I was most proud of! As most of us remember, when we think back to our early twenties, we feel indestructible, immortal, strong and fearless! Now here I was, five weeks from a massively important event for me, feeling broken, weak and fearful! I didn't know what to do next, but a couple of my housemates were medics at St Mary's Hospital medical school, and they got me icing my back and taking anti-inflammatories. Two days later not much improvement was happening, and I was missing training sessions. One of my rowing buddies, Pete, casually mentioned that his brother, Neil, was a chiropractor and practiced 20-30 minutes away. What's a chiropractor, I thought? I had never heard the term before!

Anyway, Pete booked me in with Neil, and feeling cautious, curious and sore, I went along to his chiropractic clinic. What happened at the clinic was all a bit of blur. However, I certainly remember that I felt about 50% better when I walked out. Just two or three visits later and I felt great, pretty much 100%, and by following Neil's advice and being a little careful about what actions I took for a few days I made an amazingly swift recovery. I was very soon back in the boat, and fantastically, I made it to the Championships. How we got on there is a long story for another time! However, at that moment I took all this a bit for granted. I was so focused on my reason (my 'Why?') to recover and be able to compete that I didn't step back to wonder at the speed of my recovery.

My curiosity was suddenly sparked by my chiropractic experience. I returned to Neil's clinic, and he was kind enough to allow me to spend time with him, observing patients and watching what he did. What made me very excited, and this would have happened, I believe, whether or not it was 'chiropractic', was that Neil was observing, assessing, diagnosing and adjusting (the chiropractic word for manipulation of the spine and extremities) all these people who were presenting with a wide range of conditions. He also saw great results, on a day-by-day basis. My passion for chiropractic was alight!

While I was studying geology at Imperial College (my friends would say I was studying rowing) I clearly did not have the passion for that subject. I was certain I was passionate about chiropractic, but even more so about health, and what constitutes health. As a result, I went on to study, and qualify, as a Doctor of Chiropractic, a full 5-year course following on from my degree at Imperial College!

While my rowing ambitions were never totally fulfilled, I have gone on to try and fulfil them with chiropractic. While I never got to the level to trial for the GB Olympic rowing team, I did get selected as a chiropractor for London 2012! Being a member of the London Olympics organising committee's medical team was a fantastic experience. I was based at the polyclinic within the Olympic village for rowers and sprint canoeists. Funny how life pans out sometimes, isn't it?

Stop blaming yourself!

The vast majority of people I speak to are quite aware of what is 'good' and what is 'bad' for their health. However, I am always astonished by how many people I meet who are oblivious to the state of their health. If we know what is good and bad, then why are so many people overweight or obese? Why do people smoke, drink alcohol and/or eat low-quality food? Why are most people so sedentary? A common pattern is that at some tipping point you decide to take action. You then become increasingly frustrated as you go around in circles with diets, exercise binges, controlling alcohol, etc, but always end up back where you started.

Change is often put off, deferred until it will be easier at some point in the future. How many times have you said to yourself, "Next year will be my year!" What happens when next year comes? Nothing bloody happens! You go back to the same old pattern of procrastination, bad habits, and weak old excuses. So, when you want to improve your health, it is vital to know your reason **WHY** you want to improve it. For example:

- Have you had medical worries? If you have, how severe were these?

- Do you want to be able to play with your grandchildren?

- Are you unhappy, or depressed with how you feel?

- Do you suffer ongoing pain?

- Do you feel anxious about your future?

Albert Einstein was quoted as saying:

> *"Insanity: doing the same thing over and over again and expecting different results."*

The simple solution? Find a series of easily sustainable changes that you can stick to. Even if these are realistically achievable challenges for you, you will still have to work bloody hard, over and over and over again. You will have to keep up this mindful persistence for as long as you can to make these changes habitual, but most important of all is to always, always, remember your reason *WHY!* I will cover what these changes are throughout this book. Make all these changes, and your health will take an enormous leap forward. Stick to some of the points in this book, and you will benefit greatly. So, stop blaming yourself, absorb the details in this book, remember your reason *WHY* and enjoy feeling better than ever!

You have One Body and One Life! Don't Screw it Up! If this book can help just one person make a massive difference to their life, that is amazing. If not for God's sake, then for your own sake, **PLEASE make that One person be YOU!**

1

Why Is This Book Called One Body One Life?

"The first wealth is health."

Ralph Waldo Emerson

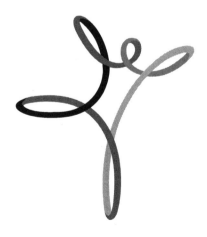

How DNA relates to your health, and what I mean by One Body One Life

First things first, don't get anxious, as I am not going to regurgitate the physiology and chemical structure of Deoxyribonucleic Acid (DNA) and start attempting to explain the genetic code! However, my reasons to link your overall health to DNA is twofold. First of all, while your DNA code is fundamental to life and creates your individual blueprint, your health is NOT written in stone, or dictated, by it. The outline of your health is controlled by your genetic makeup. This controls approximately 20% of your health whilst the remaining 80% is down to your environment.

Secondly, there has been amazing work (and Nobel prizes won for work) done looking at chromosomes. This work has concentrated on the ends of the chromosomes that are called telomeres. You can think of these structures as the tip that stops a string, rope or shoelace from splitting or fraying at the ends. Your cells are constantly dividing, with the average human body producing approximately 300 billion new cells every 24 hours. That is a massive number! Every time a cell copies itself and divides, these telomeres get shorter. Once they get too short it is impossible for that cell to divide again. This is an objective way to measure ageing, and research now shows that the length of your telomeres is a very accurate indicator of potential longevity. I will talk more about telomeres later, as we should all do what we can to minimise their shortening, and try to do what we can to get them to lengthen again!

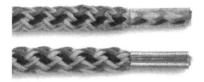

Figure 1: Shoelace "Telomeres"

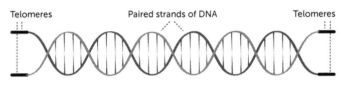

A chromosome is made of paired strands of DNA forming
a double helix and telomeres at each end.

Figure 2: Chromosomes and Telomeres

Fascinating studies have taken place looking at identical twins and evaluating their health histories over time. Have you ever known any identical twins? I have known three sets of identical twins. Identical twins will, unsurprisingly you may think, look identical! This is true until they leave home and mum. Up to this point in their lives they have grown in the same environment, i.e. they have eaten the same food, played similar sports, done similar activities, etc. Because of this their genetic expression has been the same. Genetic expression is the way that your DNA coding is expressed and how your body has responded to the outside world, i.e. your environment. Studies have looked at identical twins once they have exceeded 40 years of age. Do you think they all look similar? Do you think they all have the same medical history? The answer is a resounding 'No!' A few pairs, usually living close together, will still maintain a very close similarity. The vast majority, however, look quite different.

Imagine a pair of identical twins for a moment. Twin A has gone off and eaten fantastically for 20 years, exercised daily, stayed in a mobile job and been proactive with their health. Does s/he look very different to Twin B who sits at a computer all day, only eats fast food, smokes heavily, drinks too much alcohol or fizzy drinks, is a stress cadet and last exercised six months ago? I hope you will agree that if Twin B repeats that lifestyle for 20 years, then their health history will be vastly different, and not for the better.

My belief, after 18 years in chiropractic practice, is that the vast majority of people take their health for granted. I think it is completely natural to feel immortal (as I did when I was rowing) when we are young. We do not accept, or understand, however, how much we can control, and influence, our future health by our actions today. Parents also owe a duty of care to educate their children. We cannot expect public health to improve if we have forgotten the basics of good health! We owe it to ourselves, our families, and our communities, to live our lives in a state of our best possible health.

One Body One Life is the code to maximising your health, so that you can live feeling happy, healthy and well. I want as many people as possible to not 'just survive', but rather to 'Feel Alive!' Your lifestyle and environment will dictate how fast your cells will age. This can be visibly seen in the length of the telomeres at the end of every chromosome, in every cell in your body. Whilst it is unlikely that you will get to have your cells analysed in this way, what will you do to minimise ageing and maximise your health potential?

What is Health?

I believe a fantastic, accurate and practical way to assess health and the risk of future health issues is based on the physiological concepts of allostasis and allostatic load. What's that you ask? Allostasis describes how your body and mind adapt to environmental stressors. These may include internal stressors, such as the loss of spinal function, emotional stress and ongoing, low-grade, stress responses, and external environmental stressors, such as unhealthy lifestyle habits, unhealthy home or work relationships or a polluted environment. These stressors may lead to adaptive changes in your gene expression. Allostatic load is due to cumulative wear and tear on the body, the measure of the amount of accumulated stress the body and mind systems are under due to chronic, persistent and repetitive stress. The longer both your body and your mind are exposed to these chronic, stressful, loads from your poor lifestyle habits, then the more likely the adaptations will occur. Adaptations in neural (nervous system) or neuroendocrine (nervous system and hormonal) responses in your various body systems will eventually lead to illness.

Does that last paragraph seem a little bamboozling? If it does, let's simplify it and look at how we age. We usually judge ourselves along very strictly chronological lines, i.e. as every decade passes we seem to feel changes compared to the last. Take yourself back to when you were about ten years old. Your body was elastic, your energy was amazing and you slept like a baby. If you climbed a tree and fell out, you would probably cry out of shock, and about five minutes later, when you had dried your eyes, you were getting back up into that tree! Now, if your Great Aunty Winnie (bless her) had climbed that tree and fell out, there is a good chance that she is not getting back up again! This is because when you are ten your body is built out of 'rubber and Kevlar', the body is elastic and has a very large range of tolerance before reaching a point that gives pain and discomfort. Poor Great Aunty Winnie's body is not elastic anymore. Her range of tolerance is very small, and in fact if she has constant discomfort from, for example, an arthritic hip, then there is a zero range of tolerance in that particular joint because it has worn down to that severe level of change.

You may feel that this is common sense, but if we continue to judge things in a purely chronological way, then a twenty-something should always be able to do things that an eighty-something cannot. The last time I watched coverage of the London Marathon, there were a good number of runners who had completed the race and were over eighty years of age! Wow! Yes of course there were many, many more runners competing who were in their twenties and thirties, but there are also millions of people in their twenties who could not even consider starting a marathon. So, in this oversimplified model, who is healthier and living with better function? The eighty-year-old marathon runner or one of the multitude of people in their twenties who cannot run to the end of the road?

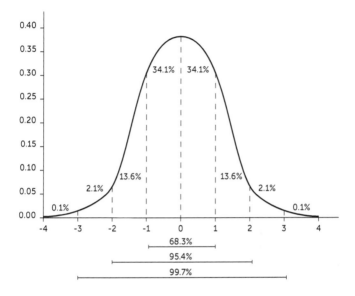

Figure 3: Normal Distribution curve

Now, a normal distribution curve like this image can demonstrate what the most common occurrence is within a population and that there are also exceptions to the rule. We can see these exceptions at either end of this curve. There will always be exceptions to this rule, but as a population we distort what we perceive as normal. For example, being obese is now extremely common but being obese is never normal. High blood pressure is ridiculously common, but again, this condition is never normal. The majority of the population's perception of healthiness is very common, but is not correct, and we even know the main reasons why! Too many calories ingested, too few burned off. Far too much time spent being sedentary, and this is getting worse by the generation. Laptops, tablets and smartphones are all too compelling for today's younger generations. I am certain that we will see the trend of obesity, Type 2 diabetes, raised blood pressure (hypertension), stress levels, back pain, etc, steadily continuing to rise *unless* public health continues to improve. The general public must become better educated to take responsibility for their health, and be incentivised to take charge of their health, before they screw it up!

The generation who grew up in the aftermath of the Second World War did everything better than we did bar one thing – they smoked much more! Otherwise, that post-war generation were much more active, grew up on simple rationed food, did not drink anywhere near as much alcohol and had a slower pace of life. Yes, life was more austere at that point in history, but only a tiny fraction of the working population was sitting for a living. In the USA or UK today the most common profession is being a *'professional sitter'* because whether you are a lawyer, accountant, IT consultant or whatever, you still sit full time for your living.

As long ago as 1948, the World Health Organization (WHO) defined health as "a state of complete physical, mental, and social wellbeing and not merely the absence of disease or infirmity".

I feel two things about this definition are amazing. First, isn't it fantastic that this was defined in such a way back in 1948? The inclusion of physical, mental and social aspects to creating a state of 'wellbeing' was forward-thinking. Second, why do the vast majority of people I meet feel that their healthcare is now reactive, allopathic (symptom-based) and not able to look at the whole person?

I promise not to overwhelm you with technical terms, but I do want to briefly explain homeostasis. In the human body homeostasis means a condition of stable equilibrium of all systems in the body, especially those maintained by our physiological processes.

Health then is purely a state of consistent homeostatic cell function. This is the normal state for the human body. Anything other than this is not health, and is therefore a state of dis-ease, i.e. the precursor to disease or symptomatic problems.

Your Environment Dictating Health

I believe that approximately 80% of our health is down to environmental factors, while the remaining 20% is dictated by our genetic makeup.

Let's deal with the genetic side first. It seems to me that you can barely get from one week to the next without the scientists finding the 'this' gene or the 'that' gene. Listening to the news tends to make people feel that virtually *every* aspect of their life, and health, is being controlled genetically.

Now, please don't get me wrong. Clearly, a lot of diseases involve many genes in very complex interactions, and these will be affected by environmental factors (discussed later). It is very rare to be born with certain forms of cancer, heart disease or diabetes, for example, and most babies are therefore healthy. Some of these babies may be at high risk of acquiring a specific disease though, and this is called genetic predisposition.

Let's think about cancer for a moment. Many studies have shown that major lifestyle factors, such as poor diet, a sedentary lifestyle, and tobacco use are much greater determinants of cancer risk, rather than inherited genetic factors. However, a few types of cancer, including the inherited BRCA1 gene, account for a very small percentage of people who (like Angelina Jolie), if this gene is detected, do indeed have a high risk of that disease. However, this is no guarantee that breast cancer will develop. The behaviour of this gene, like any other, can be turned on and off by correct nutrition, relieving mental stress, exercise and an overall lessening of the toxic load upon the body.

The Curve of Life

I like to make things highly visual when I can, and I explain the concept of ageing (inevitable to all of us I am afraid) by way of this diagram:

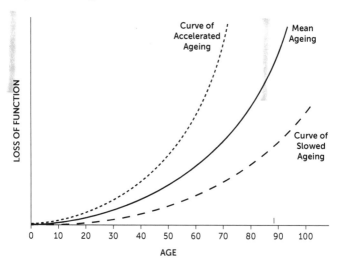

Figure 4: The Curve of Life

You can see age along the bottom of the graph and functional change up the side of the graph. Functional change represents loss of normal musculoskeletal function, wear and tear, apparent dis-ease and worse disease, pain and weakness. All of this means that we have moved away from a state of consistent homeostasis!

So, what does the graph tell us? Well, barring trauma, most of us are perfect when we are born and still perfect at ten years old. By twenty we clearly should still be functioning very well and our bodies are very tolerant to stressors. However, commonly I see young people present to me with loss of spinal function due to sedentary posture and time on their pads, pods and screens!

By thirty we know, however fit we may be, that we are not twenty any more. By forty we know we are not thirty any more, and so it goes on. The speed of functional loss continues to speed up exponentially as we get older. The projected line of this curve is pre-ordained by our genetic code, but how it pans out is, at the very least, 80% affected by our behaviour, life events and environment.

To give an example of how the curve is affected, let's think back to that pair of identical twins I asked you to imagine earlier. Do you remember them? Good. So first think of Twin A. He has eaten fantastically for 20 years, exercised his body daily, stayed in a job that allowed him to move around (or at least stand) and been proactive with his health. Doing all of these things consistently will slow the curve, and you could produce a dotted line extending out below the initial curve as his lifestyle is slowing the rate of change.

Now to Twin B who sits at a computer all day, only eats fast food, smokes heavily, drinks too much and last exercised six months ago! I'm sure you will agree that Twin B's line, in all likelihood, is going to extend out above the initial curved line drawn, and will curve faster, suggesting that he will age faster.

Other factors can also affect the curve. Twin A could be living their life, when they are involved in a severe road traffic accident, leaving them with multiple broken bones and trauma. Could this type of event leave an indelible mark on their function and health? Yes. But this event could also have happened to Twin B. If this was the case, which of the twins would you expect to make the faster, and better, recovery?

Is There a Perfect Environment?

Can there ever be a perfect environment? Well, that depends on what you will define as perfect. But it is clear that there are many straightforward factors that will be explained in the coming chapters about improving lifestyle contributors to our environment.

But this has to be a practical solution! Too many people know that their lifestyle is 'out of whack', they feel that their health is not what it should be, but they feel under immense pressure to just survive from day to day. Commuting to work, holding down the job to pay the rent, ferrying the kids to and from school, etc, etc. The pressures of modern-day life lead us to rely on releases such as alcohol, tobacco, binge television-watching and fast food. These give us a quick fix by changing our biochemistry. Sadly, their overuse will lead us down a path away from health.

The Myth of Life Expectancy

Is your perception that average life expectancy is lengthening or shortening? Most people would say that it is lengthening, yes? Life expectancy in a country such as the UK or USA is approximately 77-78 years. But are we actually living longer, and with a good quality of life?

A life expectancy average is a funny thing. Imagine a world where half of all children born die on the day of their birth, but the other children all live and pass away on their 100th birthday, living an active life right up until that day. What is the life expectancy of that world? 50 years. Anyone who survives their first day will live a full and active life until the ripe old age of 100. Does this demonstrate accurately what is going on in that society?

Returning to our world, we know there is strong evidence that way back in the pre-industrial or pre-agriculture eras our ancestors lived very full, long and active lives as long as they avoided death from lack of food, childbirth or fighting! As time moved on and societies began developing large towns and cities, we saw life expectancy plunging due to terrible sanitation and spread of disease caused by the close proximity of people. We then figured out how to distance ourselves from sewage in the streets and develop agriculture to raise food standards. The availability of clean water also improved, and as these improvements in living standards established themselves, so the average life expectancy started to extend once again. It is believed that life expectancy, in Tudor London, was in the mid-twenties!

There is now an increasing weight of research suggesting that while the average life expectancy in the West is 77-78 years, the average person will only be able to enjoy about 65 years of good-quality and fully-functional life! So, on average one sixth of our lives is spent with a poor quality of life. Modern medicine has demonstrated a great ability to prolong the lives of people who have poor health, but it has not shown any ability to improve the baseline health of the older population and increase the functional lifespan. Surely we would all rather enjoy, and should demand of ourselves, as high a quality of life as possible, for as long as possible?

Rather than looking to modern medicine for the answer, more pressing should be the following two questions:

1. What does your body need to function correctly and promote health?

2. What factors are toxic to the body, cause dysfunction and adversely affect your health?

In the following chapters I am going to discuss the Functional Health Pyramid. This will explain the way I look at three main contributing areas to health of FRAMEWORK (your neuro-musculo-skeletal structure), FUEL (everything that enters your body via food, drink or absorption) and FEEL (all factors affecting your mental health). But I would like to introduce you to some vital concepts now.

What does your body need to function correctly and promote health?

Your body needs to have a strong structure, in the same way as a building must have strong foundations to build upon. In the human body, the foundations, your FRAMEWORK, are your central nervous system (the brain and spinal cord), skeleton and muscles. Our amazing bodies evolved over many hundreds of thousands of years. We evolved into hunter-gatherers and lived in tribes. We were always active. The men were out hunting or protecting the livestock while the women went out gathering fruits, roots and herbs, looked after the children along with the elders, and prepared the food. These people never, or only very rarely, sat on their bottoms. They would squat for long periods while preparing food, for example, or they would be walking. Your body has evolved to be walking for about 15-20 km per day, along with the occasional sprint, climb, heavy lifting, and of course the occasional fight!

As such your body is designed to be mobile and flexible. Your body is designed to sustain being challenged and stay strong. Your body needs to maintain spinal and extremity joint mobility. You should also keep good muscular strength.

The FUEL your body craves should be straightforward! It is not fast food! Your body will thrive on natural food, eaten in a pattern similar to your hunter-gatherer ancestors. Fruits, vegetables, nuts and some meat or fish when available. The body also needs to be well hydrated.

How should you FEEL? I'm not going to tell you that those hunter-gatherer ancestors of yours had it easy each and every day, but they were living congruently with their environment. They were in balance. They would get up at dawn and go to bed when it got dark. They lived in balance with nature and thrived and survived. They had time to be calm as well.

What factors are toxic to the body, cause dysfunction and adversely affect your health?

The toxic patterns to the body are those that we see all too commonly today in the western world.

Your FRAMEWORK is challenged by our overwhelmingly sedentary lifestyles. How common is it for patients of mine to follow a typical daily pattern of: get out of bed, drive/train to work, sit all day at work, drive home, sit in front of the TV, get back into squishy bed, wake up, and repeat?

Sitting for prolonged periods, over months and years, will inevitably cause distortion of posture and lead to an anterior head carriage. Every 2cm that your head is further forward than it should be causes the relative weight of the head to increase by 50%! So, let's assume your head weighs 4kg. At 2cm anterior to its ideal position it will feel like 6kg to your body. 4cm anterior to neutral equates to 9kg, and 6cm anterior to neutral equates to a whopping 13.5kg! This is more than a three-fold increase in weight, and 6cm anterior to neutral is a very common position to find the head of desk-based workers.

This distortion pattern creates a reaction in the body, and starts to increase stiffness. Poor spinal flexibility leads to irritation of the joints and stimulation of nociception (pain causing) receptors. When stimulated, this releases cortisol and catecholamines (stress hormones) and these create a pain cycle.

Recent research has also reinforced the link between sedentary life and the increase in the prevalence of knee arthritis. Whilst the excuse for the increasing cases of knee arthritis was increasing life expectancy, it is now strongly believed to be down to problems associated with our modern lifestyles that have become ubiquitous. This is primarily an alarming lack of movement!

What toxic FUEL do we load our bodies with? When it comes to food in the western world in 2018 it has barely ever been cheaper to buy calories. We commonly see that the most calorie-rich food is usually the cheapest, for example, crisps, chocolate, chips, cake and fizzy drinks. Have you ever tried to see how hard it is to cut sugar from your diet? It is hiding everywhere, in breakfast cereals, in stir-fry sauces, and in vast quantities in many soups and drinks.

We also eat loads of 'white' food, by which I mean white bread, pasta, rice, potatoes, which are all very rich in carbohydrates and high in calories. We consume vast amounts of high fructose corn syrup which is used to prolong shelf life and sweeten food. Man-made trans fats are also used to prolong the shelf life of many baked goods. It is an extremely long compound that when it gets into our bodies it actually stiffens cell walls affecting their basic function.

Also included in this section is what we absorb, actively or passively, into our lungs or through our skin. Tobacco, industrial pollution, and chemicals from many products applied to the skin, all have clear health implications for us.

What factors that change the way that we FEEL can be toxic to us? Well, first let's remember the link between physical stress and mental stress. They are inextricably linked. Now, I am no mime artist, but what would you do physically to demonstrate the emotion of anxiety? You would probably clench your fists, shrug your shoulders, stick out your chin and grit your teeth together! So, a series of physical actions demonstrate an emotion, because this is what many people are doing on a daily basis. "I am stressed!" We hear this all the time. If you are not convinced, let's think of two people. First, just imagine a world-class athlete the day before competing at a major athletics event, at the peak of physical fitness after years of training. If they were suffering from severe anxiety, is it likely they will perform at their peak? No chance. Or what about the millionaire, playboy son of a Russian oligarch who is living on his dad's motor yacht in Monaco, surrounded by a group of beauties. Life is pretty good, but if he has chronic pain, is it likely he will be very happy? No chance of that either!

Stress, anxiety and depression, let alone any more serious mental health challenges, will all have a toxic physical impact on the body as well as a mental effect.

Are You Feeling Alive Now?

How are you feeling right now? Do you feel happy, healthy and well? Are you *Feeling Alive?* Or rather, how are you currently expressing your DNA, that makes up your unique set of blueprints? We are about to explore the three factors,

Framework, Fuel and Feel, that make up the overall Function of the Health Pyramid. To do this we need to assess some baseline measure, and examine how your health may be being expressed if you are not Feeling Alive.

All the time remembering you have One Body One Life, I want you to change habits so you don't become another statistic of someone who has screwed up their life by being blind or ignorant to the truth in front of you!

2

Stress:
A Modern Pandemic

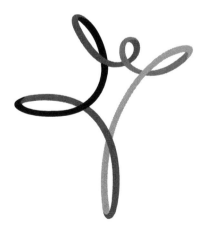

Stress is such a commonly used word nowadays, but this is not a surprise to me as we are overloaded with it! We are exposed to it in the three forms of physical, chemical and emotional stress.

Research studies have linked stress to the shortening of the telomeres at the ends of your chromosomes. One remarkable study examined two groups of mothers. One group contained parents of normal healthy kids, while the second group cared for very poorly children. Quite scarily, the care-giving mothers had telomeres that appeared 10 years shorter than those of the other group. You read that correctly: the cells of the stressed mothers were behaving as if they were the cells of people a whole decade older than they actually were! So, this pandemic of chronic stress that surrounds us is not just about people being in a grump. Stress contributes to accelerated ageing, and the effect is significant.

Our evolved physiological reaction to stress is brilliant when seen in the environment that it is evolved to respond to. Imagine one of our caveman ancestors walking through a jungle, followed by his/her young children. They enter a clearing, and as they do they see an enormous tiger appearing at the other side and it is staring at them intently. This results in an immediate stress response! The body triggers a fight-or-flight response, essentially a sudden release of adrenaline into the blood. The effects of adrenaline are to raise blood pressure (by constricting blood supply to the stomach, intestines, kidneys), increase heart rate, increase blood supply to the heart, lungs and muscles (by dilating their arterial supply) and open the airways in the lungs. Adrenaline also enlarges the pupils in the eyes and maximises blood glucose levels to your brain. The effect of this response? You feel that you could turn and run faster than Usain Bolt, climb a tree, or stand your ground with your spear and protect your kids!

Luckily the tiger turns its back and pads off into the jungle. Phew! If this happened, the caveman's stress response would settle down quickly, and about 30 minutes later everything would be back to normal, basal levels, again.

The trouble for those of us living in the modern, urban jungle is that we are constantly living with elevated levels of stress, and this has a specific, and predictable, effect on our bodies. What are some of the most common reasons to present to a medical doctor?

- Hypertension (high blood pressure)

- Irritable bowel syndrome (and other bowel symptoms)

- Back complaints

- Diabetes

- Depression

- Migraines and headache

All of the above conditions, and many more, are directly linked to prolonged, elevated stress levels and the direct physiological response to these. It is imperative that we make changes to how we look after our bodies and what we put into our bodies, and how we go about our work-life balance if we want to improve quality of life and public health and reduce the burden on primary health provision.

My Dad was born in 1914, at the outbreak of the First World War. When he was 25 World War Two began, and he and his wife Jean had their first child, my brother Richard, in 1942. At about this stage he waved goodbye to Jean and Richard and set off for the Continent, and eventually the invasion of Italy. Occasionally he received a letter. One informed him that Jean was pregnant, a few months later another letter made it to him to announce the arrival of a daughter, Gillian. At the end of the war, and his arrival back at Victoria Station in London, in 1945, as he was de-mobbed, he disembarked from the train and made his way up the platform. As soon as Jean saw him she pointed Dad out to Richard who, apparently, set off at a furious run to jump up into Dad's arms. Unsurprisingly, the little girl hiding behind Jean's legs was a lot more uncertain about this man she had never seen!

Why tell this story? Well, many years later Jean passed away, leaving Dad with my other sister, Lizzie, who had arrived sometime after her siblings and was still very young. He worked hard, and like the majority of his generation, he smoked like a chimney. When he met my Mum he still appeared very fit for a man in his fifties. However, when my Mum was about six months pregnant, carrying me, Dad suffered a huge heart attack. He survived, but I never knew him as a father who could run around or go on bike rides. He had to be very careful, and had another heart attack when I was 13 years old. Despite stopping smoking immediately after the first incident, the damage had already been done.

Dad had had a very stressful life, like many of that war-time era. I truly cannot imagine leaving home for a war zone, unsure if you are ever going to return home, not seeing your young family for years, then re-adjusting to civilian life, losing a loved partner, working and coping as a single parent, all the while smoking, etc, etc. Was it any wonder that he had a heart attack in his fifties?

The irony is that now, in 2018, stress levels in western countries such as the UK and USA are higher than ever. Whilst most of us cannot imagine surviving conflict, there were many aspects of life in post-war Britain that were MUCH BETTER for people than today. Times were austere:

- Food was rationed, so obesity was uncommon

- Fast food did not exist; most food was home cooked

- Most people commuted to work by means of self-propulsion: by foot or bicycle

- Most children walked to school

- We drank much less alcohol

Really, the only thing that was worse at that time was the much higher level of smoking.

The Effects of Stress

The effects of stress are many, and vary in individuals. Some of the effects are very common. Sadly, I find there are many cases of misunderstanding of the difference between those things that are very common, and normality. For example, low back pain is very common but is never normal. Obesity is very common but, again, is never normal.

Ongoing stress is now extremely common. Many of the effects of ongoing stress are extremely common. THIS IS NOT NORMAL! It is completely abnormal. Here are some of the most common physiological effects of stress:

- **The musculoskeletal system**: Stress will instantly cause an increase in muscle tension, and this will not relax as it is a form of guarding. As a chiropractor, I commonly see this response leading to back pain, cervicogenic and tension headaches.

- **The cardiovascular system**: Chronic stress is a definite contributor to severe overload on the heart and vascular system. A persistent stressed state will cause ongoing raised heart rate, and this along with high levels of stress hormones in the blood will lead to hypertension, heart attacks and stroke.

- **The endocrine system**: Persistent stress is governed by the autonomic nervous system. The hypothalamus stimulates the pituitary gland to release stress hormones, predominantly adrenaline and cortisol. This is all part of the fight-or-flight response mentioned earlier, and causes a rapid rise in blood sugar levels. However, if this response is chronic, blood sugar levels remain too high. People already with Type 2 diabetes will be at great risk, while those in a pre-diabetic condition (due to obesity or genetic predisposition) are put at great risk.

- **The gastrointestinal (GI) system**: Chronic stress reduces blood flow to the GI tract. This is combined with a neural agitation of the gut that can lead to common symptoms of irritable bowel syndrome, indigestion and heartburn, changeable gut function with constipation or diarrhoea, or more serious conditions like stomach ulcers.

- **Male reproductive system**: Chronic stress can lower the levels of testosterone production, which can affect male fertility levels. Erectile dysfunction also commonly occurs.

- **Female reproductive system**: The menstrual cycle can be affected, causing dysmenorrhea and irregularity of the cycle. Also, as with men, ongoing stress can often lower libido and sex drive.

- **Effect on mood**: It is known that by-products of the major stress hormones can lead to mood changes and depression. These by-products are thought to be acting in a similar way as sedatives.

- **Effect on teeth**: Teeth? What? People exhibiting stress are the most common to be grinding their teeth (bruxism). As a chiropractor I often have people referred to me by dentists, or by word of mouth, for jaw pain and ongoing teeth grinding. (Sufferers should also visit a specialist dentist for a night splint to protect their teeth.)

- **Effect on sleep**: This can be an ongoing cycle because most people who know they suffer from stress report a poor quality of sleep. Research has suggested that poor sleep quality can be a contributor to heart disease, diabetes and weight gain. However, is it poor sleep that does this or just a correlation of what we have already described?

Prolonged stress will clearly have an effect on our mental health as well, affecting both the individual as well as their nearest and dearest. And remember, chronic stress has an objective, and adverse, effect on the speed of ageing as seen on telomere length in every cell.

As mentioned already, some stress hormones can create by-products that act as sedatives on the body, and these will lower both physiological functions as well as mood. The greater the degree of stress sustained, the more of these by-products are created. So, in cases of ongoing, severe stress, they can be a significant contributor to a prolonged feeling of poor energy or depression.

Whilst it is clearly quite normal to feel both highs and lows emotionally, we are not robots after all, and it is abnormal to suffer a persistent feeling of depression.

The symptoms of depression are a wide-ranging spectrum, but severity may move from fatigue and sleep issues along with irritability, rising in more severe cases to feelings of hopelessness and, at the very worst, suicidal thinking.

Both the physiological and mental effects of stress will contribute to social effects as well. Constant pain and discomfort, or persistent mental strain, will lead to anger and irritability. A sufferer will inevitably lash out verbally, and often the first to feel this is their family. At my chiropractic centre, I commonly hear from clients how they are struggling to cope with an overload of stress, or that their partner is. People are desperate for help. The most common 'solution' is anti-depressants. It is believed that about 1 in 10 adults in the United Kingdom are taking anti-depressants! 1 in 10! Like many medicines, anti-depressants may mask the symptoms, but will not do anything to alleviate the cause. The causes of depression can be physiological, chemical, mental or social, so we must learn how to identify the primary cause.

The Causes of Stress

Stress, in its various forms, challenges us constantly. The human reaction to stress is brilliant and normal, but your body cannot react positively to prolonged or constant overload of stress.

So, what are the main causes? These will be expanded on further in the Health Pyramid. However, I summarise these causes under three headings:

- Framework: stress to your physical structure. This may be due to factors such as poor posture or overload due to obesity.

- Fuel: stress due to chemical overload. This may be due to factors such as poor food choices, but also what we absorb into our bodies through our lungs or skin.

- Feel: stress from mental anxiety, depression and social causes.

Stress in the Workplace

It appears very common to be extremely stressed in the workplace, so common in fact that it is now accepted as the norm. The particular types of stress that challenge are dependent on the type of work that you do, how much you love the profession you are in, and factors away from the workplace. Let's think of some of the common factors, though, in terms of Framework, Fuel and Feel in the workplace.

My Spinal Health Centre is based in Reading, Berkshire. Reading is a town with a high level of people in technical jobs, as well as many making the commute to the City of London every day. As a result, I see a huge number of people who are 'desk drivers'! It doesn't matter whether you are an accountant, IT consultant, airline pilot or administrator, as these types of profession, and many others, are all sedentary. We are simply not designed to sit for hours on end with minimal exercise or mobility. It is not just the seated professions that are the problem. Most professions are very specific: you train to do a very niche role. For example, a brain neurosurgeon may stand for hours on end, very still, looking through a microscope as they work, keeping their neck flexed all the time.

Drivers don't escape the mechanical overload either. Car seats are worse than desk chairs. This is because they cause your lower back to flex, rounding your spine into a C-shape. The seats in heavy goods vehicles and the like are not so bad, but the drivers of these vehicles are absolutely sitting for a living! I have seen many coach drivers presenting to me as a chiropractor, all with the same story. They have arrived at either the destination hotel or airport, and have to leap out and open the boot. Reaching into the boot, with that long hook they have, they stoop and bend to drag the suitcases and holdalls towards them. Bang! Sudden, severe, mechanical strain on overloaded discs and joints. It is the 'perfect storm' for a low back injury, or even worse, a prolapsed intervertebral disc.

How about our diet while at work? Now don't get me wrong. Some people are really good about their diet at work. A simple breakfast before they go, a packed lunch and water bottle with them and possibly some fruit for a snack. However, how common is it now to see coffee shops and fast food outlets in town and city centres? How many 'buckets' of latte and cappuccino are drunk daily? How many chocolate bars, crisps and cakes are eaten as convenient snacks between meals? I find that it is common to think that many sugary drinks, such as Lucozade, are considered healthy due to their marketing. The levels of obesity and rapid rise of Type 2 diabetes do not lie.

Many of us are feeling the increasing pressure of workload. Companies are demanding ever greater productivity whilst job insecurity increases. Pressure to hit deadlines and workplace bullying leave many people feeling isolated and insecure. On top of this we have to co-ordinate childcare, the school run and the daily commute. This is why you can feel like you have done a full day's work just by the time you arrive at work!

Stress at Home

An Englishman's home is his castle! A very true statement, and for many of us home is where we feel most comfortable. Sadly, though, many people suffer a stress overload at home as well. And for some, home can become a prison of its own.

From the structural perspective, the greatest problems at home are poor seating and levels of exercise. Sleep quality is another big issue. We should be aiming to achieve 7-8 hours a night of good-quality sleep and feel refreshed upon awaking. A poor quality of sleep affects many systems, particularly the brain. It is estimated that 1 in 3 people suffer from poor sleep. It has now been demonstrated that prolonged poor sleep significantly increases your risk of obesity, diabetes, high blood pressure and heart disease. Prolonged poor sleep will certainly lead to anxiety and depression.

Many people are brilliant at healthy home cooking, and this has been helped in recent years by the rise of the inclusive TV chefs such as Jamie Oliver. The flip side of this is the huge numbers, particularly younger adults, who struggle to know how to cook even a roast chicken! The lure of ready meals and take-aways is too much for many. This food is cheap, easy, and packed full of calories. It's also packed full of bad fats, sugar and salt.

I believe that the area of greatest stress at home is usually in the Feel area. Even in the strongest and happiest of relationships we have our challenges. Managing home and career and surviving the stresses of the kids growing up is tough. But many people have things harder. As relationships struggle or break down, maybe leading to divorce, stress can become extremely high and hard to manage. If someone is already struggling, then an overload of stress like this will escalate other health issues, as well as lead to an increased risk of escapism in the form of, for example, alcohol or drugs.

Loneliness and social exclusion also raise our stress levels. Loneliness is a terrible burden for anyone; it's a black hole that most find very hard to escape. We are naturally drawn to groups, and enjoy the company of others. Becoming withdrawn from others will, nearly always, lead to depression and anxiety. Clearly, some people do thrive on their own, but these people are usually very spiritual and have chosen this way of life as a conscious decision. They are often admired because they are quite rare, and this is because most of us would not find it easy.

Stress and Ageing

Ageing is, of course, inevitable. However, it is my observation that the majority of people believe that the manner in which they age is inevitable. I have already stated my belief that this is untrue. Do we all get older? Yes. Will some people age better than others? Yes. But we can control this process significantly. Please cast your mind back to the normal distribution graph I described earlier. The actions that we take can allow us to predict the usual outcome. However, there are always exceptions. For example, one of my longstanding guests at my Spinal Health Centre is a lady who is 90 years young. She has smoked between 30-40 cigarettes a day for about 70 years, so I hope she had shares in one of the tobacco companies! She seems as fit as a flea! But this is not usual. Most people who smoke heavily will reduce their lifespan and their quality of life very significantly. We know this to be true. Likewise, I know of young people very sadly passing away from lung cancer despite never having smoked.

The two examples above indicate those people at either end of a normal distribution graph indicating lifespan and smoking or not. I feel the need to demonstrate this point because it is absolutely true that some people may live a very healthy life and yet very sadly succumb to some disease that takes them away far too young. The converse is that for every one of these people there is someone who seems to defy the odds. This person may be smoking, drinking heavily, making poor food choices leading to obesity and still living to a ripe old age. Is it fair? No. But there are many factors that we can control, even into old age, that can improve our health, and the numbers of years that we enjoy good health.

Framework in the elderly:

Look around you at elderly people. Look at their posture. What do you see? Are they, on the whole, very upright or bent forward? I would say that they are bent forward. Anterior head carriage develops insidiously as a slow repetitive strain injury. This develops almost always as a result of too much sitting. Remember, it is common to find people exhibiting anterior head carriage of more than 6cm and this results in more than a three-fold increase in relative head weight.

Anterior head carriage is an obvious sign, but is part of the greater danger of overall poor spinal movement. I remember a wonderful patient who I knew for about four years whilst in my first chiropractic position. His name was Frank, and he was about 80 years young when I first knew him. He used to cycle to and from the centre, about six miles each way, for his monthly chiropractic checkup. Quite often when I checked him there was nothing for me to do, so I would send him on his way without asking him to pay. I kept encouraging him to come monthly though, to ensure that he was staying loose, and he thought that was great. Frank would not get his daily paper from the local shop, no, he would cycle three miles the other way to get it and run errands for his neighbours. He also loved gardening, and would garden for several of his even more elderly neighbours to keep their homes looking shipshape. He told me he never watched television but would sit in the evening to read or listen to the radio, and that he would be on his feet pretty much all day until he'd had his evening tea.

Is it a coincidence that Frank was still so active, fit and strong? I don't think so. Likewise, I have seen videos of Japanese masters of Kung Fu who were doing the splits and handstands. These men were in their 80s. Had they just started doing this? Not a chance. They had been practising their art for their whole lives and had maintained this function.

Research has now demonstrated, unequivocally, that our personal environment, especially physical inactivity, accounts for the majority of chronic health conditions. We can consider inactivity to be less than 30 minutes per day of brisk walking or an equivalent exercise. Indeed, it appears that these factors may make up to 80% of the causal factors in three of our most common health afflictions: coronary heart disease, Type 2 diabetes and many location-specific cancers.

Poor posture from sitting too much, and non-activity, over an ongoing period of time will be devastating to anyone's health. We know that low levels of mobility lead to loss of function at the spinal level. This leads to pain signals being sent to the brain which has been shown to affect neuroendocrine, muscle and autonomic nervous system function. At the same time there is a decrease in healthy motion inputs required for healthy neuroendocrine, muscle and autonomic nervous system function. A double whammy!

This continued lack of motion is most commonly seen in the elderly. Sadly, this is now being seen in young adults as well as we get ever more sedentary. Structural decay occurs with loss of spinal function, and leads to accelerated degenerative joint disease (osteoarthritis) as well as osteoporosis.

In my opinion, regular chiropractic care, spinal mobility exercises and strengthening work are just as important for spinal health as regular dental hygiene is in maintaining your teeth. My poor grandma had her last tooth pulled out at the age of 24 (in 1924). We would be horrified at this happening today. And yet as a society we still find premature arthritis to be acceptable or normal. It is NOT normal! If everyone was as proactive about their spinal health as they are (for the most part) about their dental health, we would be much, much healthier!

Let us not forget those genetics again though. Some people are going to be more prone to bone wear and tear than others. My own Mum, for example, needed a full hip replacement while she was still in her 50s. She had not suffered any trauma, ate a good diet, never smoked, and had been a busy working mum. So why did her hip wear out too soon? Mum has naturally lower bone density (lower on that normal distribution curve), and after I had qualified I noticed that she has very overpronated feet, meaning that they roll in. This overpronation leads to overload and will cause the hip to rotate in as well, leading to increase in wear and tear. I believe that, had this been noticed earlier, then her hip would have lasted longer due to decreased load.

Fuel in the elderly:

As we get older we tend to get less active. Rare exceptions, such as my former patient Frank, are still active into their later years. However, the majority become very sedentary, and this at the same stage of life when our metabolisms are slowing down means that we need fewer calories to maintain our energy expenditure. Sadly, the majority of older people are overweight, and being overweight in our latter years is even harder to deal with than when we are young.

The food equation is very simple. If your calorific intake is in excess of your needs, you will put weight on, and if the balance is the other way, you will lose weight. A full day every day of sitting in your chair does not require many calories, and yet people fail to realise this.

A dear friend of mine, Nicki, is a community nurse in beautiful Cornwall. I know that she enthuses passionately all the time, and tries to help and educate her patients as much as possible. Sadly, she sees a similar pattern very commonly in the elderly. She told me of one lady who was housebound, in fact she was pretty much chairbound. Being very obese she was also wearing incontinence wear as she could not

49

move fast enough to get to the toilet in time. She had a 24-pack of crisps on one side of her chair and a large bottle of Lucozade on the other, as this was a "healthy drink". When my friend pointed out to her that this was not the best, or most nutritious of combinations, she said, "But eating crisps is one of the only things I enjoy". Nicki didn't bother to point out that it was this kind of behaviour over many previous years that had led to her predicament now. This leads on to the Feel section.

Feel in the elderly:

The case of the lady described in the previous paragraph is clearly not only about food, but about how she was feeling about herself. She was very depressed, as well as challenged by what she ate. She was clearly also challenged by a severe lack of movement.

I am a firm believer that you are only as old as you feel. If you can run a marathon over the age of 80, it is rare and amazing, and you are probably physically fitter than the majority of twenty-somethings who would have no chance of completing that marathon.

I know a wonderful lady called Sylvia. She has previously been a patient of mine. Sylvia is a full-time home support carer. She is lean, fit and full of energy and the joy of life. She chats constantly, whenever I see her, about her family, especially her grandchildren. She loves her job and loves caring for people. I asked her if she was planning to retire at any stage. She just laughed at me, saying, "Why would I retire? What would I do? Do you want me to just sit and watch television? My brain would rot in five minutes and

I would be bored senseless. No, I will work for as long as I can as it keeps me healthy." These were her words with no prompting from me. She is an inspiration to me, and her vibrancy speaks for itself. She is still living with purpose, at 72 years of age, and certainly has no intention of doing otherwise. Many people of a similar age wake up in the morning, have breakfast, and then sit in front of the TV all day, every day.

A lot of elderly people become isolated and lonely. This social exclusion is a common cause of great stress as well, further worsening concurrent physiological issues.

Stress Busting Tools

1. Exercise. This is massively important. Exercising regularly will produce neurotransmitters that act as natural anti-depressants. They also have an action of decreasing muscle tension in the body. This does not have to be complicated. Get out of the house and walk. The very best walking coach is a dog!

2. Good Food. Simple: eat good food. Cut out all the artificial stuff, eat less, drink less alcohol and caffeine. Try to eat so that you are a 'hungry wolf' and not a 'podgy bear'. Do not follow a fad diet. You need to change your manner of eating and maintain it.

3. Meditation and Mindfulness. Spend time outside in nature and focus on breathing. Meditation is something I have tried and have struggled with a lot. My mind tends to spin along at a million miles

per hour. However, this does not need to be scary. You just need to chill out. You can find guided meditation that only takes 10-15 minutes to do if you are really busy, or use other equipment such as BrainTap which I will refer to later.

4. Emotional Freedom Technique (EFT). EFT is a form of acupressure that you can use on yourself. We know that emotional health is essential to both physical health and your ability to heal. Even if you positively challenge stress to your Framework and Fuel, you will not relieve your mental stress if you do not remove your emotional barriers. EFT can be used to reduce negative emotions, reduce your bad food cravings and reduce pain you are suffering. You can find details of how to learn and implement this online.

I will give you more specifics on these tools as I break down the steps further.

Chiropractic can help reduce your stress

Now I want to explain a little about the structure of the nervous system in relation to how chiropractic helps. The cerebellum is the part of the brain that receives all sensory information. It is sent all this data from sensory organs, the spinal cord and other parts of the brain. The cerebellum is the area that coordinates your posture, balance and speech.

The vermis is the area within the cerebellum that becomes stimulated by spinal movement. Chiropractors believe that specific chiropractic adjustments improve mechanical function and improve the neural function from the brain to the body, and the body back to the brain.

At the most basic level though, Chiropractic is about motion and mobility. An ever-increasingly large amount of evidence is reinforcing the importance of correct spinal function to our physiology and good health. We also know that correct spinal mobility sends proprioception (information about our joint position) signals to the vermis. And we also know that incorrect spinal function sends nociceptive (pain) signals to the vermis.

Chiropractic adjustments increase the movement of a joint by removing the mechanical restriction. This allows normal function of the vermis so that all other sensory information to the cerebellum can be understood and ensures that normal physiology occurs as a result.

Chiropractors are primary health care practitioners. Medical doctors are fantastic at what they do, but they look at the body depending on what the symptoms tell them. They work in a sickness and disease paradigm. Chiropractors look at the body holistically, meaning that they look at the body as a whole, and try to understand how everything is working in relation to everything else. They work in a health and wellness paradigm.

A chiropractor may well become the first point of contact for a person in the management of their health. Don't get me wrong; there are certainly times when you may need to consult, or be referred to, your medical doctor.

3

The One Body
One Life Pyramid

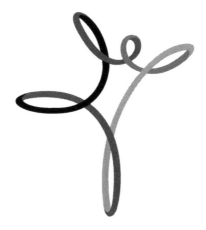

What is the premise of the One Body One Life Pyramid? It is to understand and counter the fact that we are living sedentary lives, eating vast quantities of a toxic and nutritionally-deficient diet, and living under emotional and spiritual overload.

The One Body One Life Pyramid is a model of functional health, a combination of the three constituent areas of Framework, Fuel, and Feel. It is a model that everyone can commit to. You do not have to be a saint all of the time and neither do you have to be like Jane Fonda doing your exercises in leg warmers and sweat bands!

I do believe that as many people as possible need to fully understand the elements that contribute to overall function, health, and wellbeing.

How does the model work?

The three elements of Framework, Fuel and Feel all contribute equally to overall function. You may be great in two of the areas, but a significant weakness in the other will lead to loss of overall function.

For many years I was a professional rowing coach as well as a chiropractor. I coached to a high level including at the Junior World Rowing Championships and the Oxford-Cambridge University Women's Boat Race. There were clearly three elements to being an excellent rower: technique, physiology, and mentality. You could see an athlete who had amazing physiology (a strong engine) and fantastic technique (the ability to move the boat efficiently) but was soft mentally. Despite their potential to move the boat, they would not live up to their potential unless this area was improved. Likewise, you could find similar patterns with a weakness in any one of the areas.

Good function and therefore being healthy requires attention to all three areas or you will end up developing a reaction to that prolonged stress.

The aim is to achieve the optimal function for you, regardless of your age. While optimal function for an 80-year-old person is not the same as optimal for a 20-year-old, it is clear that most people are functioning well below their optimal function.

I will discuss each area in full in the immediately following chapters.

Framework Pyramid

"Re-Frame and Align Your S.P.I.N.E."

- **S is for Sedentary and Structure:** We know that being sedentary is toxic to the body, and mobility actually creates positive feedback to the brain.

- **P is for Posture:** Correct posture is the position in which the body works most efficiently, and where everything is in balance. Any abnormal posture, such as anterior head carriage, causes overload and accelerated wear and tear, and physical stress.

- **I is for Innate:** Innate responses are not learned or practiced. They are an automatic reaction, by the brain and body, to a specific stimulus. While the body is working in balance (homeostasis) the brain and body will respond accordingly.

- **N is for Neurological:** Our central nervous system (the brain and spinal cord) is the most precious system that we have, and is the master system in the body. This is why we protect it inside the skull and the vertebral column. Correct function of the nervous system is essential for correct function and health.

- **E is for Exercise:** We need to move! We have evolved as hunter-gatherers and must be mobile. Our evolution dictates that we should be doing lots of walking, occasional sprints, some heavy lifting and climbing and even the occasional fight.

Fuel Pyramid

"H.E.A.L. yourself from the inside out."

After all, you are what you eat!

- **H is for Hydration:** Crucial and so simple, yet most people are commonly dehydrated.

- **E is for Eat:** What food should we eat, and why? Likewise, what should we avoid eating as it's harmful to the body, and why?

- **A is for Absorb:** Whilst eating and drinking forms the bulk of what enters our body, we must also include other chemicals from sources such as smoking, air pollution, drugs (medical and non-medical) and chemicals applied topically on the skin (such as skin creams).

- **L is for Life Supplements:** Sadly, there are now an ever-increasing number of dietary supplements that we need to add to our normal diet to ensure we meet our needs.

Feel Pyramid

"F.E.E.L. Alive"

- **F is for Focus:** Focus here relates to your ability to recognise your mood, whether you are feeling low, and to take action to effect a change.

- **E is for Environmental:** How do the factors of our current life, where we live, if we are thriving or surviving, society pressures or trauma affect how we Feel and cope?

- **E is for Energy:** The mind is one of the very biggest contributors to energy levels so mental energy and physical energy levels are intrinsically linked.

- **L is for Love:** The feeling of loving and being loved, both by others and your own 'love of self', has a massive impact on our mental health which causes direct effects on pain levels and self-worth.

The Function Pyramid

Function clearly requires a balance of all three other pyramids. It is impossible to have normal function if there is a weakness in one of the other three contributing areas. Technically, when the body is functioning well it is in homeostasis, i.e. all these elements that govern the body are in balance and equilibrium.

Just remember to "Re-Align the S.P.I.N.E., H.E.A.L. yourself from the inside out and F.E.E.L. Alive!" If you do that you will be in great shape.

One Body One Life – Don't Screw It Up!

4.

The Framework Pyramid - Re-Frame and Align your S.P.I.N.E.

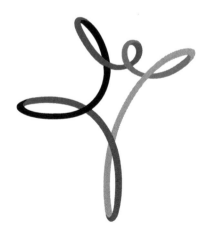

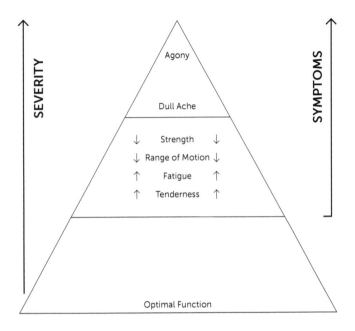

Figure 5: The Framework Pyramid

The framework pyramid is a model relating to the neuro-musculo-skeletal system, i.e. your nerves, muscles, and bones. At the base of the pyramid is optimal function, and the range that I consider normal is the bottom third of the pyramid.

The top third of the pyramid relates to subjective symptoms, i.e. those symptoms that most people are aware of, so this will be pain. The very top of the pyramid will be 'agony', whereas at the bottom of this section the symptom may be a 'mild ache'. This is clearly a non-linear scale as there are many points in between agony and a mild ache.

So, what is the section in between? This relates to objective symptoms. These symptoms are ones that many people may not even be aware are present until a practitioner tests them to demonstrate the problem. They may be symptoms such as decreased strength, loss of range of motion of a joint, increased fatigue and tenderness to touch. This is not a complete list, but a selection of common objective symptoms.

Why are these important? To many people they may not represent an issue. However, I have worked with Olympic athletes and professional footballers. If you are an Olympic athlete, do you need to be at your absolute peak performance level for the duration of your events at those games? Absolutely! The vast majority of professional athletes who I have had the pleasure to work with are not in pain. Having pain at the Olympics would be a disaster for an athlete, as it is highly unlikely that they will be able to perform at their very best. Now, if you are an accountant (I am not picking on accountants here) and you are spending most of your day sitting in front of your computer, I believe it is fair to assume that you are not pushing your body to the limits of your performance. There is some slack in the system, so IF you were exhibiting many of these objective symptoms, in the same way as the athlete, it is highly likely that you would be completely ignorant of them.

The average person, when I have asked them, is honest enough to say something like, "Pain is bad, no pain is good". What they are saying is they believe that pain is binary, on or off, and that the presence or absence of pain is the absolute indicator of a problem. This is an incorrect assumption! The presence or absence of pain is not, never has been, and never will be an accurate indicator of function of the neuro-musculo-skeletal system! Prolonged presence of objective symptoms indicates irritation of the system and moving towards a worsening of the strain that leads towards pain.

Traumatic events will move you from optimal to agony very fast. For example, an elite athlete may severely sprain their ankle, damaging ligaments and muscle. This really hurts! The ankle swells up fast, throbbing pain will continue, and hardly any weight can be put upon it. However, the natural history of this type of injury is not to be a permanent one, and the pain will recede over the next 7-10 days. Will they be ready to run in 10 days? No. Will they be walking with a limp still? Yes. Eventually, there will be no pain on normal activity, but the ankle will still feel unstable and weak. At this point this injury will be in the middle section of the pyramid. I hope this example gives you clarity as to how this is a dynamic model.

It is essential to have a great framework

Just take a look at the physical form of elite athletes from any physically active sport. Both male and female athletes look great and clearly function extremely well. When your body has a great framework, you are demonstrating that your body is in balance, and that your posture is correct. This allows your body to work in the most efficient way, requiring the least amount of energy to maintain that posture and placing the least mechanical load upon the structures of the spine and extremities.

A poorly functioning framework will usually lead to less activity, due to physical symptoms that will become inevitable with poor mobility. What are some of the most important outcomes for skeletal health if we lose function of our framework?

Degenerative joint disease (aka osteoarthritis) is seen as an inevitable outcome of getting older. This wear and tear most often occurs in weight-bearing joints. This degeneration will inevitably lead to a loss of function. Loss of function, especially as we get older, leads to weight gain and obesity. Once obese, there are the other inevitable increases in risk to cardiovascular health, diabetes and other common conditions.

What about our children who are at the other end of the age spectrum? Is it reasonable to assume that children are less active now than a generation ago? There are ever increasing temptations from electronic devices, and less readiness to allow our kids freedom thanks to the 24-hour news stations' tales of constant threat in our neighbourhoods.

It has been demonstrated that regular and strenuous exercise is vital for our children. They should all be lean, strong, fit and full of energy. There should not be any child who cannot fit this model, barring those born with challenges. Children who are carrying too much weight are usually suffering from too much love from parents who sincerely believe they are being kind by not saying "No!" The benefits of regular and hard exercise for children include the formation of strong and healthy bones as well as influencing how their bone structure develops, a brilliant example of genetic expression in action. An inactive child will not load their bones, leading to less bone density being developed, and increasing their fracture risk in later life!

An Introduction to S.P.I.N.E.

"Re-Frame and Align Your S.P.I.N.E."

- **S is for Sedentary and Structure:** We know that being sedentary is toxic to the body, and mobility actually creates positive feedback to the brain.

- **P is for Posture:** Correct posture is the position in which the body works most efficiently, and where everything is in balance. Any abnormal posture, such as anterior head carriage, causes overload and accelerated wear and tear, and physical stress.

- **I is for Innate:** Innate responses are not learned or practiced. They are an automatic reaction, by the brain and body, to a specific stimulus. While the body is working in balance (homeostasis) the brain and body will respond accordingly.

- **N is for Neurological:** Our central nervous system (the brain and spinal cord) is the most precious system that we have, and is the master system in the body. This is why we protect it inside the skull and the vertebral column. Correct function of the nervous system is essential for correct function and health.

- **E is for Exercise:** We need to move! We have evolved as hunter-gatherers and must be mobile. Our evolution dictates that we should be doing lots of walking, occasional sprints, some heavy lifting and climbing, and even having the occasional fight.

The spine is the pillar for our whole body. We see during the development of a human embryo that the very first structures that become differentiated are the primitive brain and the spinal cord. From this point the nervous system starts to develop. Eventually 31 pairs of spinal nerve roots grow and branch out from the cord. The body, in its infinite wisdom, decides that it needs to protect this. So, the next thing that happens is that the skeletal system develops. First, a series of bones join together to form the skull. This is followed by a stack of 24 vertebrae that form a column, each one separated by a mobile disc. At the base of your spine is the large sacrum, which forms part of the pelvis.

If there is an irritated nerve, or what we may call a '**subluxation**', which means a bone out of place that causes neural irritation, it changes the physiology, or how an organ or body part functions and works. If there is an irritated nerve involved, not only can a chiropractor or osteopath help neck and back problems but also any number of organic problems. And when you're dealing with chronic pain that has been developing over many years, not only do you develop pain in your back, which is a classic symptom, but you may often develop some loss of function in your organs, and restrictions in the nervous system. That is why you are asked on the clinic history form about your digestion, bowels and breathing, etc.

This is often why, when a person has a neck problem, they also develop numbness and tingling in their hands and fingers. They may develop headaches. They may also develop respiratory problems. When we get to the very low back and chronic low back conditions, one of the most common things we ask is if there are any changes in bowel and bladder habits. These are very common. Organic problems often begin in the back or spine and end up affecting the organs, and again we may be able to help these conditions.

This explains my acronym of S.P.I.N.E. The spine and skull protect the most precious system in your body, the central nervous system. While the cells of other systems in the body are constantly being replaced and renewed, the central nervous system has to be protected. It cannot be replaced because we would lose our long-developed, fine motor skills, language and memories. This is why conditions such as stroke are so devastating, as medical science does not yet have an answer for this level of damage. Whilst the effects of a stroke are usually devastatingly fast, the effects of chronic overload and strain to our Framework may be insidious and incremental until such point as pain starts and the level of damage becomes apparent. It is much easier to be proactive and prepare for the future whilst living life to the full now!

S. Structure and sedentary life

The first 'S' is for structure. While I have no intention of giving you a thorough breakdown of our anatomy, I feel it is extremely important to explain a little of what forms our functional structure, and how structures work with each other to allow us to move. The key structures are bones, muscles, ligaments and fascia. You will also see that one of the fastest ways to weaken or effect adverse change onto these structures is by being sedentary, the second 'S'.

The body is designed so that we can defy gravity. It is believed that the vast majority of the computing power of the brain is being used to help us do this and remain standing. This is why it still appears very hard for robotics experts to recreate anything that looks like normal human walking. For the body to work correctly it has to be in correct posture and be aligned vertically.

Bones: The bones form our skeleton. Two or more bones create a joint, and at least one muscle crosses every joint so that movement can be created and controlled. As we move, the bones act as levers. Bones are not dead, and in fact the marrow within the big long bones is where new blood cells are produced. All bones are being replaced and renewed constantly. The largest bone is the femur, your thigh bone, and in adults every cell in the femur will be replaced and renewed every 7-10 years! As children we create more bone than we replace as we are growing. The cells making bone are called osteoblasts, and those that break down the bones are called osteoclasts. As adults this action is balanced, but as we get elderly the clastic action starts to be greater than our ability to replace with new bone and as a result our bones get weaker.

This weakening of bone is inevitable as we age, but there are things that we can do to help maintain it. Think for a moment of an astronaut circling the Earth in the International Space Station. They are floating around in zero gravity, so there is minimal load put on their skeleton because they are not having to defy gravity. Within just a few days in this environment the astronaut starts to lose bone density, and if they are in space for several months they may lose up to 20% of their entire bone mass.

Women lose a significant amount of bone after the menopause. Most women do not realise that they can lose up to 20% of their bone in the five years post menopause. This makes post-menopausal women at much greater risk of osteoporosis (weakening of the bones) and of getting bone fractures. Think about some of your elderly relatives. The majority of elderly people are extremely sedentary. Being this sedentary is very similar to being in the space station. There is less load being put upon the bones, and yet bones need to be challenged to stimulate what osteoblastic (bone growth) function that they may still be capable of.

I will talk about bone more when discussing Exercise and Nutrition. However, I will ask you this. In the UK, what is the most common medical 'solution' for decreased bone density? The answer is the prescription of calcium carbonate, better known as chalk. Well, firstly, I know that eating some chalk is not going to magically make my bones stronger without other action. Would the astronauts get stronger bones in space by eating chalk? No, of course not. Secondly, there are many minerals involved in bone development, and concentrating on calcium supplementation has been shown to increase the chance of developing osteoporosis. Thirdly, we need to look at Vitamin D and Exercise. There is a shocking deficiency in Vitamin D now, mostly due to not getting enough sunlight, but Vitamin D is vital for bone health as well as many other systems in the body. Exercise is vital, and must be weight-bearing exercise as it is essential that you stimulate the osteoblasts into action and create more bone.

Muscles: We have over 600 muscles in the human body. Every muscle crosses at least one joint, and some cross many joints. Like most constituent parts of the body they work at their best when we are young. Muscles respond to loading, and get stronger if stimulated. Did my favourite action hero, Arnold Swarzenegger, develop his massive muscles by sitting at a desk all day and in front of a TV at night? No way, he was down at the Gold's Gym pounding out hundreds of sets of dumbbell lifts. I am not recommending that you become a bodybuilder, but my point is that, if your muscles are exercised regularly, they will get stronger. Sit around all day and they atrophy and weaken quickly.

Exercise is vital to maintain muscles mass and strength. It has been demonstrated that the process of strengthening your muscles also changes hormones, enzymes and your blood chemistry so that your chances of developing many of the diseases linked to a sedentary lifestyle are significantly lowered.

Ligaments: These are considered to be pretty passive structures normally, and they run from bone to bone. Ligaments are one of the slowest healing structures in your body as they have no direct blood supply. Think about your favourite sports stars. If a footballer breaks a bone, they can often be up and about running again after 6-8 weeks. However, severely strained ligaments, for example in the knee, may take months to heal and rehabilitate, and often the player is never quite the same again.

Anterior head carriage due to prolonged sitting is caused over time by creep of the ligaments in the spine so that some are lengthened.

Healing takes time, and requires sparing from further excessive load. Most ligament injuries from overload strain will heal by about three months after the injury, as long as the excess strain has been removed.

You can think of ligaments as behaving plastically. Imagine the plastic ring that holds together four cans of beer. If you play with this and stretch it, there is a small amount of give before the plastic starts to deform. Once it has deformed it will never return to the original state. Now, your ligaments are very robust, but if they are overloaded they will also suffer from plastic deformation. Thankfully though, our ligaments do have the power of recovery and can heal if they are given the chance. However, this process will take a long time.

Fascia: This is the component that you are least likely to know about. It is a mesh, the natural fabric that holds our body together. Fascia is present throughout the body. In the abdomen, for example, fascia is the material that prevents your intestines from sloshing up and down if you are jumping. It surrounds every muscle in the body to allow smooth movement of one muscle over another. However, fibrous adhesions are formed in the fascia, either as a result of trauma or as a result of prolonged strained and postural deformation. Fascia is also very variable in form from extremely light, almost purely collagenous, in areas such as the face or breast, to very tough in the sole of the foot – the plantar fascia supports your body weight every step you take.

As with other structures in the body, the fascia will adapt to your function and motion. If you are flexible, active and varied in your activities, you will retain fantastic mobility. If you are inactive, sedentary and repetitive in the types of function that you do partake in, then the fascia adapts. This adaption will insidiously stiffen you up. This is another reason why spinal mobility exercises, or Pilates and yoga type exercises, can keep you feeling loose.

The second 'S' is for Sedentary. This is simple: as a modern society we must move more, much more than the average person currently does. Whilst there are many preventative health factors, such as obesity, smoking, drinking and social factors, I believe that our sedentary lifestyle is the number one risk factor to health, and here is why.

Multiple research projects have been done looking at the benefits of moderate exercise on various aspects of health. Moderate exercise was defined as brisk walking. So, what were some of the benefits?

- Knee Arthritis: a group which exercises three times per week for one hour each time reported a 47% improvement in their knee pain.

- Hip Fracture: in post-menopausal women regular weekly exercise reduced the risk of fracture of the hip by over 40%.

- Depression: even with very low levels of exercise, levels of depression were reduced by about 30%, and these improvements were shown to improve further as the exercise levels increased.

- Risk of Death: one study, that has been tracked over many years, has shown that those who regularly exercise have a significantly lower risk of early death than those who are sedentary.

- Diabetes: regular exercise has been shown to reduce the risk of developing frank diabetes by as much as 50%.

- Overall Quality of Life: regular exercise has been demonstrated to be the single most powerful contributor to improving an individual's quality of life.

In one huge study of over 50,000 people in the USA it was shown that a low fitness level is the highest single predictor of death! This single factor was a higher risk than hypertension (high blood pressure), diabetes, smoking or alcohol intake.

A 2017 study by Public Health England shows horrendous results for inactivity. The study included over 72,000 subjects, equal numbers of male and female subjects between the ages of 40 and 60. Just over 41% of these people failed to walk more than 10 minutes continuously, once, each month, at a brisk pace. Brisk walking was defined as "walking continuously for at least 10 minutes in the past 4 weeks and the effort was enough to raise breathing rate or make you out of breath or break sweat". Can you imagine our hunter-gatherer ancestors only managing to do this once per month? No! They would do much more than this every day! Again, can it be any surprise that our population is getting fatter and fatter and that rates of disease such as diabetes, cancer and heart disease continue to skyrocket?

The double whammy in this large study was that the combination of low fitness and obesity created an exponential rise in risk to health. Exercise was also shown to be the most powerful factor because the study also demonstrated that if someone is obese, but is physically active, then the risk to their health is significantly reduced.

Right at the start of this book I said that it is important to know that putting the building blocks of good health in place is achievable for everybody. The minimum exercise levels that you should do are not big and scary, and you don't have to be at a gym to achieve them, unless you want to. A large study done by a Japanese company of many thousands of its employees looked at the effect that walking to work had on blood pressure. Those who walked for under 10 minutes showed no change in blood pressure levels. Those walking between 11 and 20 minutes demonstrated a 12% reduction in levels of high blood pressure, and over 20 minutes showed about a 30% reduction in levels of high blood pressure. Isn't that fantastic?

I will expand on other exercise recommendations later in this chapter at 'E' for Exercise.

P. Posture

Everyone is born with the potential for perfect posture, so that includes you. Pretty much every child exhibits fantastic posture. Here in the UK this is true up until their 5th year of life. Why their 5th year of life? Well, in that year we send them to school. As our children start school they develop new habits and their day-to-day activity changes. They start being made to sit for large amounts of the day at tables, or cross-legged on the floor looking up at the teacher.

Unhealthy postural patterns are another pandemic. All unhealthy postural patterns will cause physical stress on the body, in line with the degree of postural distortion. If you have a perfectly aligned posture then you should be extremely happy, because you are a rare individual! Posture is certainly linked to back pain. It is well known that at least 80% of people will suffer from an episode of back pain at some point in their life.

There is shocking evidence of the effect of poor posture even in children. An American study of several hundred early teenage children took magnetic resonance images (MRI) of their low backs which showed that over one third of them had degeneration of at least one lumbar disc! If kids already have this damage when they should be still developing and 'practically perfect in every way', then they have little chance of being pain-free as adults.

Studies on older adults have been equally shocking. As previously stated, one of the most common indicators of poor posture is anterior head carriage. Whilst the link between this and physical pain is clear, due to the exponential rise in load as the head translates forward, this posture also has effects on organ health. Anterior head carriage can reduce lung capacity by up to 30% which can lead to heart and pulmonary disease. A rise in blood pressure, leading to hypertension, can also be linked to posture. This is due to a neural connection between the muscles in the neck and the nucleus tractus solitarius, which is a part of the brainstem that controls blood pressure.

Common Causes of Poor Posture

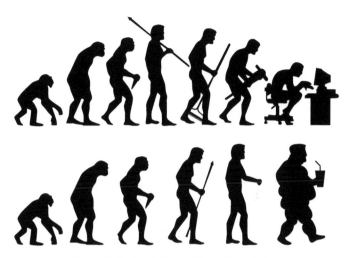

Figure 6: Postural change through evolution

Whatever your age you can affect your posture, for good or bad. However, in a postural sense, have you seen that we only seem to get more bent over as we age? More alarmingly, however, there is a greater prevalence of younger people presenting with fixed, bent-over postures. Our ape ancestors used to be bent over, but we developed from quadripeds to bipeds. As we evolved we became ever more upright, lean and muscular. Now, we are getting more slouched again, hunching over our desks and computers, getting ever more sedentary and overweight. Our environment is changing much faster than we are able to adapt to it, and as a result our bodies are suffering. This suffering results in adverse health reactions.

So, is it possible to simplify how our posture is affected? Here are five of the common posture-affecting factors:

- Our sedentary lifestyle: Every part of us, whether joints, muscles or nervous system, requires daily mechanical stimulation. I have already explained how immobility causes bone loss and muscle weakening and increases stiffness. As this becomes prolonged, these initial changes will stimulate conditions such as osteoporosis, degenerative joint disease and permanent loss of normal posture.

- Anterior head carriage: Associated with too much time sitting down, this also causes the mid-back to round forward into a C-shape. Inevitably, the shoulders are pulled forward, the sternum drops and compresses the heart and lungs, and muscles adapt to this. Some muscles become short and tight while others are weakened.

- Stomach sleeping: A pet hate of mine, yet one that is so common. If you sleep like this you are twisting your spine severely, as your head will be turned to one side and usually you will have one hip hitched right up.

- There are two good sleeping positions. The first position is on your side, knees slightly bent. If you have any low back pain, then place two pillows between your knees as well, as this will reduce the mechanical load on the low back. This is also a great help to ladies in their final trimester of pregnancy and can give them a comfy night's sleep. Alternatively, try sleeping on your back, but ideally with the knees supported in a slightly bent position. A shaped memory foam pillow is also highly recommended to keep the head and neck supported in a neutral position.

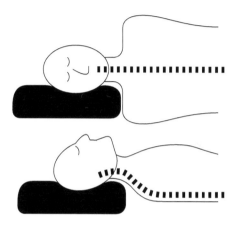

Figure 7: Neck pillow support diagram

- Abnormal foot mechanics: I find it hard to believe how many people have presented to me with back pain, and therefore poor posture, who have never had their feet looked at. They may have seen medical doctors, physiotherapists, chiropractors or osteopaths before, but never had their foot biomechanics assessed. Overpronation (the foot rolled in), a collapsed arch in the foot, or poor shoe choice can all cause severe postural change. After all, if a building has terrible foundations, do you fancy staying in the penthouse suite?

- Repetitive movements and bad lifting: The majority of jobs require us to perform the same activity over and over again. This repetition creates adaption, and frequently overuse. We can see similar adaption on a lady wearing an excessively heavy bag on one shoulder, and always the same shoulder! A warehouseman will be unloading pallets, and usually bending and twisting in the same direction for many lifts. Either of these examples leads to asymmetry of the skeleton and muscular imbalance.

Why is Good Posture Important?

Let's start with our children. Our kids develop many of their lifestyle habits while at school. The remainder they pick up from the behaviour of their parents and what they learn from various media sources. If children develop poor postural habits at a young age, it is almost inevitable that these will persist into adulthood.

Academic performance and occurrence of back pain are related. This demonstrates the need for postural education in schools, which is something which is very lacking at the moment. Back pain is worryingly common in school-age children and studies have shown that those with such pain suffer academically.

A common cause of posture change is a child wearing an overloaded rucksack or backpack. It has been clearly shown that no child should be carrying a pack that weighs more than 10% of their bodyweight. The majority of children are wearing backpacks that exceed this suggested limit and overuse injuries are far too common.

Typically, children are sitting for around 6-8 hours per day at school. If you get a chance, have a look at how your child, and their classmates, are sitting. I suspect you will see them slouching, round-backed or slumped down over their desk. It will be rare to see them sitting upright and alert.

I believe that children and adults should be using a foam wedge cushion on their seat. This seat wedge is usually angled at 11 degrees and makes it easier to keep your pelvis in the correct position.

In adults, incorrect posture can alter performance by decreasing and adversely affecting the structure. Maintaining a good posture can decrease fatigue and raise your mental state. This especially relates to neck function. A well-aligned spine that is controlled by strong and balanced muscles will also prevent low back pain and maintain better balance in older people.

Can bad posture be the cause of an early death? Yes, it can. An excessive curve forward in your mid-back has been shown as a predictor of death in both male and female subjects. If you lose over 3cm in height due to poor posture, you are much more likely to die because of a heart attack.

Do you run a business? Does the posture of your workforce affect your bottom line? The research suggests 'yes' to this as well. Studies have shown that companies that introduced ergonomic programmes and posture advice to their staff showed a clear improvement in increased production, less sick days due to pain and fewer injuries reported.

Are You Sitting or Slouching?

In all the world's advanced economies the majority of the workforce sits for a living. As we now know, prolonged sitting will increase your chance of developing conditions such as cancer, heart disease and Type 2 diabetes. There is no doubt that prolonged sitting can make you sick and injure you. Within just one hour of sitting damage begins in the discs in your spine. A recent study actually found that even if you exercised every working day, for about an hour, this would not be enough to counteract the adverse effects of sitting at your desk for a typical 8-hour day. None of our hunter-gatherer ancestors were sitting for this amount of time, so our bodies are not evolved to do this. It makes us sick, and significantly affects how our bodies react to this physical stress. This directly relates to our genetic expression as mentioned previously.

The spine is so vulnerable to the excess loads of sitting that it can only tolerate this for about half an hour. After this time the soft tissues, including the intervertebral discs, that sit between our vertebra, begin to absorb the extra load, leading to delamination. This is why I always recommend microbreaks when sitting. Standing up, even if only for a minute or so, reduces load. You do not have to leave your desk, just stand up every time you pause for thought. Can you stand whilst on the phone? The good news is that regularly altering your position can really help. Even if you do sit for hours, regular microbreaks as I suggest can massively help to reduce the chance of injury.

One Body One Life TIPS

I do not know who coined the phrase, "Sitting for your spine is like sugar for your teeth", but it is accurate and memorable. If you are occupied in work that requires you to sit, what can you do to improve your workspace?

- If you work at home, or have the ability to individualise your working space, then get yourself a sit-stand desk. These are ever more commonly available. Most models have electric inverters in the legs to raise and lower the desk. I love mine, especially as I am about 6 feet 6 inches tall. When standing, it is perfect, and when I do sit at it, the ideal desk height for me is much higher than the standard desk height.

- If you are not in a position to stand at times, then get yourself a good chair. The chair needs to be adaptable in height so that your feet are flat on the floor while your hips are higher than your knees. The chair base should be tipped forward so that the front of the seat is lower. If your chair does not do this, then you must have a seat wedge that does the same thing cheaply and effectively.

- I believe that sitting back onto a chair will guarantee that you are slouching. I have seen evidence suggesting that the seat has to have a well-controlled lumbar support, but I do not buy this. My experience suggests that those who suffer back pain need to learn to control their posture with their core muscles, and that relying on a chair to control you is a very short-term solution. A correctly angled seat base should allow you to maintain a neutral, upright pelvis, leading to a neutral spine that you hold off any back support.

- Your computer screen should be at your eye level, straight ahead of your eyes. This is one of the key reasons why 'hot desking' is so bad. This work pattern usually means working with a laptop. A small keyboard and low, small screen cause you to lean forward and stoop your head down. If you work from home and have to work on your laptop, then a great tip is to buy yourself a full-sized USB keyboard and mouse, and place your laptop on about 5 or 6 hardback books (or enough to ensure that your screen is at eye level). This allows correct screen height and comfortable hand position, and you will have a greater chance of maintaining a good position.

- Further to the previous point, you should maintain a good position for your hands, wrists and elbows. A correct height of desk and chair, along with full-sized keyboard and mouse, should allow for a good position. Prolonged wrist extension can stimulate carpal tunnel syndrome, which is due to persistent irritation of the median nerve as it passes through the wrist.

- Take regular microbreaks. Standing up at your desk at least every 30 minutes, for about 30 seconds, can pay massive dividends. A great exercise for this break is the Brügger Exercise. Stand tall with the palms of your hands facing forward, arms straight down but about a foot away from the sides of your body. Pretend someone is pulling them lightly backwards and down. Raise your sternum (the breast bone) and retract your chin. Do not look up or down here but try to make a double chin. Then take in a deep breath and let it out slowly. Repeat. This fabulous exercise makes you switch on all of the muscles that are normally being stretched and inhibited by poor sitting posture, and stretches those becoming short and tight.

Posture From The Ground Up!

Everyone would recognise the famous Tower of Pisa. It is unique because of the way it leans over. Is the top of the tower the problem? No, the problem clearly lies with the foundations. In the same way, your feet are the foundations of your body. However, the vast majority of people have never had their foot, ankle and lower limb biomechanics assessed.

Each of your feet is made up of 26 bones, and if you count the two tiny sesamoid bones under the ball of the big toe it's 28. The function and alignment of your feet can significantly affect your whole posture. The most common form of dysfunction is overpronation, which means that the feet roll in to the midline too much. If you have significant foot overpronation, you may be knock-kneed, suffer discomfort in the arch or sole of the foot, may have pain farther up the leg and you may notice that your shoes are wearing down faster on the inside rear corner of your shoes. Whilst there are various forms of overpronation that I will not expand on here, the type and severity may lead to other symptoms such as mechanical back pain.

If you are sporty and enjoy high impact sports, such as running or tennis, overpronation may lead to additional issues in your feet, ankles, knees and hips. These issues can include common conditions such as shin splints, plantar fasciitis, Achilles tendonitis and the development of bunions.

When a patient of mine asks me about their bunions, I usually chuckle when they tell me, "My Mum has bunions so I must have got them from her". Well, when was the last time you saw bunions on a baby? Never. You inherit looks from your parents, hair colour and eye colour, but not bunions. You will, however, inherit similar foot mechanics. As a child you may be overpronated but not demonstrate any symptoms because of how tolerant your young body is to physical load. Bunions are a result of consistent overload in the joint which forms the ball of the big toe. It is a form of premature arthritis. If that excess load is reduced, sooner rather than later, then the bunion formation can be halted.

When I see this very common set of symptoms in the lower limb, I am always going to take a very good look at the alignment of the pelvis and spine, as overpronation of the foot causes the knees and hips to roll in. As a result, the pelvis rolls forward, and this causes a cascade response in spinal function. As we have to find our balance point, the low back leans back further and then the upper back curves back forward. So, foot function can increase the curves in the spine, and increase load.

Ongoing, persistent, lower back pain is very common in people with foot overpronation. For some people exercises may be beneficial, and may affect function. These will have a chance in younger people, and especially in those who will work on the exercises daily and consistently over a long period of time. For the majority of people, the best care is to have prescription foot orthotics fitted correctly, as these will control the foot and effect structural change throughout your body.

I. Innate

What is innate, and what does it mean to you? As a chiropractor, the concept of innate intelligence is very important to me. It is the concept that your body has a natural inborn intelligence and ability to work perfectly, given normal circumstances. The ability for your body to develop, and for good health, is hardwired.

At the cellular level, look at our immune system. The cells of our innate immune system, the white blood cells, are our first line of defence against infection and cancer cells that are formed daily. The cells that make up our body have their own life cycles. We constantly create new cells, and break down old and damaged ones. Damage occurs through a wide variety of methods such as sunlight, drugs, x-rays and trauma. Damage to a cell's DNA may lead to a normal cell turning into a cancerous one, but this requires a certain amount of DNA damage. The definition of a cancerous cell is tricky though. Is it cancerous because it has damaged DNA, or has it the predisposition to develop into a cancerous tumour? Either way, our amazing innate immune system constantly identifies, hunts down, and destroys these damaged cells.

This is a great example of innate health at the cellular level. Looking at the body as a whole, we have to realise that we are designed to be healthy, and for our amazing body to work, in a healthy way, for a long time. Once again, it is our environment that is affecting us. Do you have, or do you have friends or family who have, a toddler? I love remembering my boys when they were about 18 months old. At that age they would often sit on the floor of the lounge, legs out straight with a lovely upright back. Watching them breathing, there was zero chest movement. Instead, you could see their little tummies moving in and out. They were breathing with their diaphragm.

When I assess respiration at my clinic I ask someone to take a deep breath. Well over 90% of adults will take a deep breath by raising their sternum and shoulders and lifting the whole rib cage as a result. This is panting, and is abnormal. So, why do we all pant? Once again, this is down to sitting too much.

Exercise: Stand up and place one hand on your tummy and one on your chest. Now, please try and take a deep belly breath. You should feel the hand on your tummy moving in and out but I need you to keep the chest motionless. When you can do this easily, please sit down. Now be honest and slouch as you normally sit at your desk, or in the car or on the sofa. While in this slouched position try and belly breathe. It is impossible! In this seated position you are bent forward, and the contents of your abdomen are pushing up into the diaphragm, doming it upwards. You cannot breathe correctly.

Why is this important? Respiration is vital for health. If you were suffocated, how long could you survive? For most of us it is somewhere between 30 seconds and one minute before death. Oxygen is the number one source of energy, and life, in your body. Now, while suffocation is a horrible thought, it represents a total loss of oxygenation of the body, clearly resulting in death pretty fast. However, can you live in a state of partial oxygenation? Yes, many people are decreasing the efficacy of their lungs by poor respiration.

Studies, including those by winners of the Nobel Prize, have demonstrated the dangers of poor oxygenation. Living in this state can lead to cells ageing faster, or altering in their ability to function. A study using rodents showed that ongoing poor oxygenation leads to the development of cancer.

Another system that is directly affected by poor posture leading to poor respiration is the lymphatic system. Many people are oblivious to this system until something goes wrong with it. It is a passive system and requires the body to be both well-hydrated and exercised and for you to be breathing correctly for it to work efficiently. The primary functions of the lymphatic system are to allow the movement of white blood cells throughout the body, and the transport of lymph fluid around the body. If there is no pumping action, or motion of the body, toxins then begin to build up in the lymph system, and you can think of it as a series of canals that run into disrepair. These would be sluggish, and full of rubbish! Correct belly breathing is the most effective way of stimulating normal movement of fluid around the lymph ducts, and the drainage of lymph fluid into the venous system.

So, your body is designed to work correctly through innate intelligence. In the example of the lymphatic system, it is the environment, specifically sitting down for too long, that changes our respiration and therefore has an effect on a separate system, the lymphatics.

Top-Down Inside-Out

How our amazing body develops can be seen by how we develop from the very first moments of life. At the very start there is one cell from Mum, and one from Dad, the egg and sperm. We call that an undifferentiated cell, meaning that if you put that cell under a microscope the only thing you can tell about it is that it is human. The first thing it does is divide into two. Then it divides into 4, then 8, then 16, 32, 64… and so on.

After about 16 days of life these cells become differentiated. They have identity, a unique identity, You!

The first cells whose function differentiates are those of the primitive brain and central nervous system. If you are going to build anything of any importance, you've got to have a good set of blueprints, and the brain and nervous system form the blueprint.

It is not my intention here to write a detailed account of the embryological development, but rather give you the relevant, and general, details and how these affect our innate development.

The brain continues to develop, and from there the nervous system develops. The body, in its infinite wisdom, decides that it needs to protect this. So, the next thing that happens is that the skeletal system develops. A series of 24 bones, the vertebrae, are stacked one on top of another with a disc in between. A pair of spinal nerves branch out between every single one of those vertebrae. So, first the brain and spinal cord develop, and second the skeletal systems for protection.

The next thing that you would notice starting to develop are the early signs of organ buds. The first of these to be seen is the heart. All the organs will develop in this way, as will the muscular system.

If there is an irritated nerve or what we may call a '*subluxation*', which means a bone slightly 'out of place' that causes nerve irritation and may alter the physiology, or how an organ or body part functions and works, not only can a chiropractor or osteopath help neck and back problems but they may also help any number of organic problems. And when you're dealing with chronic pain that has been developing over many years, not only do you develop pain in your back, which is a classic symptom, but you may often develop some partial loss of function in your organs, and restrictions in the nervous system.

This is often why, when someone has, for example, a neck problem, they also develop numbness and tingling in their hands and fingers. They may also develop headaches, and respiratory problems. When we get to the very low back and chronic low back conditions, one of the most common things we ask is, are there any changes in bowel and bladder habits. These are very, very common. So, many visceral problems often begin in the back or spine and end up affecting the organs.

Remember Frankenstein's Monster?

Do you know the story of Frankenstein's monster? I am sure you do. This is the story of Dr Frankenstein, who collected all the body parts he needed to make a human and supplied it with electricity to bring it to life. We all know that wouldn't work because when someone dies we say they are "no longer with us" or they have "passed away", because the life force has stopped flowing and the body is simply the house they lived in.

Nothing we can do to that body can bring it back to life. So, what is this life force? Well, we don't fully understand it but we do know that it comes from the brain down the spinal cord and supplies everything in the body, and if you cut the supply to any part of the body then that part of the body will die.

This flow of energy runs from the top-down and inside-out. For example, if you were to break your neck, would you be paralysed from that point up or down?

DOWN, of course. You only need to look at the tragic case of Christopher Reeve, who played Superman.

Or if you were to sever your spinal cord at waist level, would you be paralysed up or down?

Again, DOWN.

I want you to imagine you are 10% dead. You're still alive but 10% of the life force flowing in your body has stopped, so how do you think you might feel? Would you even perceive that you're only working at 90% of your maximum? Or might you find that your digestion is not 100% or you can't eat a large meal late at night? Alternatively, you may have some joint ache, headache or poor quality of sleep, or you may have felt run down for some time.

To understand this concept more, think of a light switch in your home that has a dimmer switch. Turn the dimmer down low. If you can imagine this light to be one of your organs, this is how your organ is functioning when you have a poor nerve supply. This is what is happening to many people, but they are usually unaware because the restriction has to be quite severe and prolonged to become symptomatic. As a chiropractor adjusts you and relieves that pressure on the nerve, the flow of energy improves and we see the function improve. The light gets brighter! When I give talks to the public I find that many people perceive health as being binary, i.e. problem or no problem: sick or well. Using this metaphor of the dimmer switch helps them to understand that the life force, or neural energy, is still getting through but is dependent on function.

Brand New Body

Have you ever thought it would be great to have a brand new body?

Well, I have great news for you! You get a brand new body, on average, about every 10 years (this is the bones), by which I mean nearly all the cells and tissues in your body are constantly being replaced with new ones. However, many parts of your body are replaced much more regularly. The intestines change their lining every 2-3 days, the lung lining changes every 2-3 weeks, your blood cells every four months and your liver every five months.

The numbers involved in our incredible human bodies are amazing. We can estimate that the average person creates about 300 billion NEW cells every day. That is an incredible 200 million cells per minute! The rate of recreation starts to slow down as we get older. Also, we start to accumulate slight errors and the cells are not as elastic as when we were younger. These slight errors are in the DNA within every cell and are associated with the symptoms of ageing.

However, there is one part of your body that is never replaced and that is the central nervous system. So, if you have 10 pints of lager this evening, the brain cells that die as a result can never be replaced. Equally, if the pressure in your spine irritates the nerves long enough and hard enough, then you will get permanent damage, which no power on earth can restore. That is why, as a chiropractor, I am obsessed with your spine and nervous system.

The reason that your central nervous system (which is the brain and spinal cord) does not constantly repair and replace itself is that you would lose your higher functions of memory, language, balance and fine motor skills. Many of these skills took your entire childhood to learn and master and this is exactly why an event such as a stroke can be so totally devastating.

N. Neurological

Having a fully functional neurological system is vital for the whole body, but especially for healthy structural function of the body.

At the very centre of our nervous system is the brain. Most people take their brain function for granted. Clearly you will be aware of your thoughts, feelings and memories. We are more likely to fail to acknowledge complicated actions such as respiration, heart rate, blood pressure or the control of your body temperature. This is just a tiny taste of the multiple systems that the brain controls as it attempts to keep all functions in balance. The human body functioning in balance is called homeostasis.

We know that the body is under constant stress, whether that is stress that is affecting your Framework (physical), from your Fuel (all you ingest or absorb) or that you Feel (mental). For the most part your brain can handle this stress correctly and respond accordingly. However, from time to time an overload of one or more of these stressors exceeds the 'envelope of tolerance' the brain and body has, i.e. where a response can be made without a loss of function occurring.

If your brain cannot communicate normally with any part of your body, then function is compromised or lost, and symptoms will inevitably occur.

For example, it is accepted that if a joint (think of one in your spine) has lost normal function or is inflamed, it will not send proprioceptive (healthy movement) messages to the brain. Instead it will send nociceptive (pain) messages.

If a muscle that is supplied by nerves at the level of this restriction becomes overloaded, we will probably end up with a damaged muscle. If the system is working normally and that muscle is pushed too far, then a normal reaction is for other muscles to support, and reinforce, the overloaded muscle to try and prevent worse damage.

Balance – A Test of your Nervous System

The ability to demonstrate good balance is vital if you wish to demonstrate great posture and a healthy Framework.

One Body One Life Test Yourself:

First of all, stand with your eyes open, barefoot, on a hard floor. Choose one leg to lift and raise that knee so you are balancing on one foot. Time yourself. Ideally, repeat this a few times to get an accurate average (it is easy to get a 'flukey' good or bad time) and then swap to the other foot and repeat. A fail is either losing your balance all together OR having to make a significant correction where you 'walk' your feet around to regain balance.

If you find that quite easy, repeat the same test, but this time with your eyes shut. Is there a difference?

I am pretty sure there will be! There is for most people.

So, what is 'normal' and what does it mean? Ideally you should be able to stand on one leg, with your eyes open, for an indefinite amount of time. With the eyes shut I expect patients to balance for a minimum average time of 20 seconds, but 30 seconds is preferable. If you are the lead dancer for the Royal Ballet, then you should find this extremely easy!

Good balance is just as important to the function of the body as joint flexibility and strength. I tell many of my clients that it is believed that the Native American witch doctors would get a brave or squaw to run along dry riverbeds in their bare feet to resolve their back pain. They would not know why this worked, but we can see how this would stimulate the nervous system, and create lots of proprioceptive feedback to the brain, as well as stimulate and strengthen the core muscles.

It is uncommon for many, or any, of us to walk barefoot down riverbeds now. We encase our feet in shoes and walk mostly on hard flat surfaces. If you were running barefoot over grasslands or on the forest floor every day, your feet would look and feel more like Bilbo Baggins' hobbit feet. The soles of your feet would be thick and leathery and the intrinsic muscles of your feet would be much stronger. These effects lead practitioners like myself to see decreased balance skills and weaker feet, which commonly lead to dropped arches and pronation (rolling in) of the foot.

Balance can be trained in people of any age, and has been shown to produce fast and effective results. Whether for the benefit of a young athlete who has recently sprained an ankle, or an elderly person who has been suffering from frequent stumbling or falls, an individual's balance has been shown to improve by as much as 200%, and this improvement over a very short 2 weeks of daily training.

If you want to try some balance training at home, then start by standing in a door frame as it is a safe place if you lose your balance. Do not try this in the kitchen where you may be sandwiched between a boiling pan of potatoes, the knife rack and the kettle!

You want to ensure that you can balance on each foot for at least 30 seconds repetitively and consistently. Once this is easy then you should move on to try with your eyes closed. Most people find this much harder. The reason is that when your eyes are open you are using your eyes and cerebellum (the part of the brain that is dedicated to processing sensory information that relates to fine movement) to send messages down the spine to the lower limbs, and these control balance. When your eyes are shut, you rely on getting feedback about your joint position (proprioception) from the muscles and joints in the feet, ankles, knees, etc. This feedback travels via the spinal cord to the brain. The brain integrates this information and sends the response back down the spinal cord. All this should happen in a split second. It is really common for the afferent pathways (those travelling towards the brain) to be a 'bit dozy'. They need to be retrained, and this can be done fast with some balance training.

Now, if you are elderly or have had long-standing balance problems (ataxia) then you may need to practice your balance training more often, for longer and over a greater period of time for changes to become obvious. The investment in time can be extremely worthwhile though, as once trained, balance will continue to improve.

Could Your Low Back Pain Be Linked to a Neurological Cause?

The answer to this is yes and no. It also depends on your understanding of the question! The two areas I wish you to consider are:

1. Where mechanical damage / irritation to the nervous system can cause symptoms, and

2. The brain and central nervous system are the master control system. Multiple structures share overlapping nerve supply, so irritation in one region may cause symptoms elsewhere.

Now, I am ignoring here back pain that is clearly of mechanical origin, i.e. back pain as a result of direct trauma to a specific level.

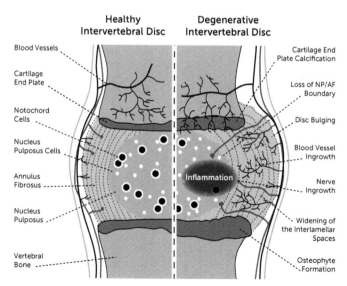

Figure 8: Normal and degenerated discs

Mechanical damage can affect our precious nervous system in several common ways. Damage to the intervertebral discs is very common and starts asymptomatically in most people. Delamination of the outer layers of the disc occurs faster as we get older. The body loses the ability to retain water within the discs. As they become dehydrated fissures start to develop in the very tough outer Annulus. These fissures usually develop from inside out, and as we move, the soft, toothpaste-like interior begins to extrude through the fissures. When this process starts to produce a partially prolapsed disc bulge the body reacts. The disc is still intact at this stage but is rather like a car tyre that you have 'kerbed' and now has a weakened tyre wall. You could still use this car if driving slowly around town (at least for a short while), but you may suffer a blowout. When a disc in the spine suffers a blowout (herniation), the material at the centre of our discs escapes into the spinal canal. This material has never been seen by your immune system as the discs were formed before your immune system. As a result, you would suffer a massive inflammatory reaction as your body would suddenly believe that an alien substance has entered your spine. This is why a herniated disc can be excruciatingly painful in the early stages of occurring.

Peripheral nerve entrapment can also cause many painful conditions. This is where there is a degree of frank neural entrapment. Symptoms may include pain, pins and needles, numbness or tingling and weakness. EMG nerve conduction studies may be used to confirm a diagnosis. If conservative management fails to relieve the symptoms, then surgery may be required to help relieve the pressure on the nerves.

Some of the most common areas to suffer a peripheral nerve entrapment are in the wrist (carpal tunnel syndrome), elbow (cubital tunnel) or around the head of the radius which is also in the elbow.

Are ALL Symptoms / Complaints Neurological?

Your body is made up of approximately 100 trillion cells. Each and every cell type within the body has a specific purpose. The function of some cells may appear insignificant on its own but groups of cells form tissue types. Tissue forms organs which in turn function together to create systems. We need normal functioning systems to allow our bodies to work normally.

Your brain is the conductor of this orchestra of systems. At a fundamental level your brain communicates and receives feedback from every cell in your body. The brain is receiving feedback and sending out messages to regulate function. As soon as a group of cells is not working properly your overall function will be sub-optimal. Clearly you would not notice this at first (as I described earlier when comparing subjective and objective symptoms), but it is inevitable that IF this loss of function continued and worsened, then at some point this dysfunction would become noticeable.

We become aware of this loss of function as 'symptoms'. Symptoms vary widely and are too numerous to list but, depending on the primary system affected, could include: pain, allergies, fatigue or asthma to name just four. If the area of dysfunction is identified, and the communication between brain and cell reconnected, then normal function may be restored.

E. Exercise

I have already made it very clear that optimal performance of your body is linked to you living as closely as possible to the way you are evolved to live. Exercise is no different. Humans have evolved over millions of years as hunter-gatherers. A normal pattern as a hunter-gatherer would be lots of walking, with the occasional sprint, the occasional heavy lifting and climbing and even the occasional fight! These activities, along with gathering roots and fruits, tending the homestead and, of course, hunting, were our primal activities. Your human body has not significantly evolved in the last 2000 years at all. We live longer because of warm homes, plentiful food and modern medicine which keeps more people alive when they get sick. However, it is our environment that has changed at an incredible rate. Do you live like a hunter-gatherer now?

As such I recommend a balance of activity that is congruent with the same pattern. We should be doing lots of exercise at a pretty easy level. This could be walking the dog, cycling or (if the weather is really bad) some light and easy cardio at the gym.

The remainder of our exercise should be a balance of high-intensity interval training (HIIT). This will include some heavy lifting, body weight moving exercises and sprinting (this could be done running, cycling, rowing machine… whatever you prefer).

HIIT exercise and other forms of increased intensity exercise will increase cell telomere lengths. A large increase in this length has been demonstrated with ultra-endurance athletes.

Now, I am certainly not recommending that everyone should start ultra-endurance training as this will challenge joints and muscles too much for most people. But this training can extend telomere lengths by as much as 75% when compared to those of sedentary individuals.

We also need to counter the dangers of being sedentary, and the inevitable stiffness that this stimulates. If you are someone who sits a lot, whether as a necessity of your job or you are retired and don't need to rush off for a job anymore, a range of simple spinal mobility exercises can be done in your own home and should be done daily. Think of them as spinal flossing. We all know that we should brush, and floss, our teeth daily. The benefits of doing that are very clear, but a lot of people fail to maintain it. You need to maintain your spinal flossing to retain normal motion as well as see your chiropractor for regular spinal adjustments.

The final area of exercise is core strengthening. By this I mean a series of specific exercises that help to strengthen your spinal stabilising muscles and improve your balance. These can also be done at home. Pilates can help people improve this and is suitable for most people. You should be careful with starting a generic Pilates course if you have been suffering from ongoing back pain, as some of the exercises may be contraindicated. I would recommend finding a local, well-recommended chiropractor or osteopath for a thorough spinal examination first.

The Benefits of Exercise

This is a massive topic and I have already mentioned some of the many benefits of NOT being sedentary in the previous section of 'S' for Sedentary.

So, what are some of the other major benefits of getting moving and really exercising your body?

- **Reduce your risk of developing Type 2 diabetes**: There are now many studies demonstrating that a combination of weight loss and moderate regular exercise will reduce your chance of developing diabetes by well over 50%. It has also been demonstrated clearly that if you are skinny but inactive, you are at double the risk of becoming diabetic than someone of similar build who is active. This makes me very anxious, particularly for the generation of young ladies whose exercise statistics are terrible.

- **Improve your cardiovascular health**: Simple, the fitter you are lowers your risk of heart disease, including heart attacks and stroke. Inactivity is also one of the biggest risk factors in developing coronary artery disease, and raising blood pressure.

- **Prevent obesity**: I have already discussed the dangers of sedentary life. Obesity levels are rapidly increasing and, in fact, obesity is now so prevalent it is retuning our perspective of body composition. Studies have shown that nationally we consume similar quantities of calories now as we did about

50 years ago. However, our populations get heavier and heavier. Why? We move less!!

- **Protect your bones**: Degeneration of the bones (often called osteoarthritis) is usually seen in the weight-bearing joints of the body, most commonly the hips, knees and spine. It is very common to find those people who suffer from severe degeneration to also be overweight, unfit and carrying an increased risk of cardiovascular disease. Regular exercise makes the joints work, stimulates the muscles around the joint, and increases load bearing through the joints that help maintain bone density.

- **Improve your brain function**: Yes, really! On the window of my Spinal Health Centre I have a quote from Nobel Prize Winner Dr Roger Sperry who said, "90% of the stimulation and nutrition to the brain is generated by the movement of the spine". Exercise helps to stimulate proprioception (normal movement stimulus) to the brain. Normal proprioception is necessary for the brain to function correctly and maintain the body in homeostasis. In the elderly, we know that a sedentary lifestyle leads to a decrease in mental skills. Brain cells only need three things, in the right balance, to function normally and thrive. These are oxygen, food and regular stimulation. As Sperry also said, "Movement is the main source of stimulation. You have to use it or lose it!"

Aerobic and anaerobic exercise

Aerobic exercise is what most of us do, most of the time, when we move. Aerobic exercise can be maintained for long periods of time as long as you can get enough oxygen. It would be practically impossible for me to overstate the multiple benefits of mild-to-moderate aerobic exercise. It is the foundation of your exercise and could constitute activities such as brisk walking, cycling, hiking or a gentle go on the rowing machine.

Regular aerobic exercise will improve your health and your quality of life, and will probably ensure you live longer, with many more years of functional life!

Anaerobic exercise is the type that you do when your body cannot get enough oxygen. If you picture Usain Bolt exploding down the 100m track, he is exercising anaerobically as he is using all his muscles maximally. Lifting heavy weights will do something similar.

As with aerobic exercise, there are huge benefits of anaerobic exercise that large swathes of the population never achieve, because they simply never do this type of exercise! As I mentioned with regard to HIIT training, our hunter-gatherer ancestors did lots of aerobic movement (mostly walking) and then the occasional sprint, heavy lifting, fighting or climbing which would all be anaerobic exercise.

"What the hell are your 'core muscles'?"

This is one of the most commonly asked questions at my centre. So, what are core muscles and why are they so important? A correctly functioning core is essential if you are sporty and want to perform to your best, and if you want to prevent injury. We know that if you have already suffered from mechanical lower back pain, then some of your key spinal stabilising muscles will atrophy within the first day or two of injury and will not regain their strength without correct stimulation.

Your spine is an amazing structure as it is 'designed' to carry the weight of your body, respond to extra load when you are moving around, and can allow you to move without looking like a robot. The 'design specs' for the spine were to encompass all the requirements of life. However, it wasn't designed to cope with excess body weight or sitting all day in a distorted pattern. Inevitably we are more sedentary now, and many people are carrying a little too much weight. Ensuring that your core is as strong as it should be, though, will protect your spine from damage.

As your spine is placed under greater and greater load you require increased strength to control the spine. I think most of us would agree that if we could have the core strength of an athlete like Daley Thompson or Jessica Ennis-Hill implanted into us, then our chances of lower back pain would be vastly reduced!

The core muscles are a group of muscles that sit in all planes around the abdomen. This is the area below the ribs and down to the top of the pelvis, including the front, back and sides. I am not going to break down every muscle type to you as I am not writing an anatomy book. However, some of these muscles are very deep and lie close to the spine while others are much more superficial, so there are planes in terms of depth of muscle also.

Whilst I have the utmost respect for many physical trainers and gym instructors, there is a wealth of misinformation swirling around about 'the core'. Much of what is still taught revolves around a few misinterpreted pieces of research from the 1990s that indicated that one or two muscles were the key players. This is wrong! It is also wrong to attempt to rehabilitate this part of the body if there are underlying issues with the inner structures including the spine, pelvis, and diaphragm.

For this reason, if you are suffering any ongoing discomfort or weakness in your back, I recommend getting this checked out by either a chiropractor, an osteopath or a physiotherapist prior to starting any form of core exercise programme.

All these aspects need to be exercised, and at my centre we commonly recommend exercises and diagnostic procedures developed by world-renowned spinal biomechanist Professor Stuart McGill, but ONLY once an individual can pass all inner and outer core competency tests. Professor McGill has done more research in this field than most and he has destroyed many of the myths associated with old training tips for the abdominal area. For example, McGill has demonstrated that 'old-fashioned' sit-ups are one of the most efficient ways possible to damage your spinal discs. He also proved that exercises that encourage you to pull your belly button in actually weaken you.

McGill has proven that you need to strengthen all planes of movement and protect the spine while you do that. Exercises on your side, on your back and on your hands and knees may be required for total core strengthening and balance.

If you are pain-free and functioning well, you should commit a few minutes every day to keep these motion patterns reinforced. If you are going to be given these types of exercise by a practitioner, then be prepared to work daily for about 15 minutes over a period of 3-4 months before they will have created structural change. I will talk more about these exercises in my programme towards the end of the book.

Can I just do Pilates or yoga?

'Yes' and 'No' would be the simple but unhelpful answers!

My first question to you is: Are you suffering from any back pain or aches and pains anywhere else at the moment? My second question is: Have you had any symptoms like these in the recent past?

If the answer is 'No' to both of these questions and you feel you wish to try either Pilates or yoga, I would give you my encouragement. My personal preference would be Pilates, especially for the beginner. As you find you enjoy exercising then you may wish to add yoga into the mix of movement.

If the answer was 'Yes', then you may still benefit from a generic Pilates course. However, again I would encourage you to consult either a chiropractor, an osteopath or a physiotherapist and get thoroughly assessed before starting anything new. Some patterns of lower back pain symptoms are suggestive of disc damage. Disc damage would be a contraindication for some exercises done in both Pilates and Yoga. At my centre we manage the spinal rehabilitation and core programme within the centre, following the McGill programme for safe core strengthening. If you are unsure, you must get checked out first. Get checked out by an expert in this field rather than your medical doctor.

5

The Fuel Pyramid – H.E.A.L. Yourself From The Inside Out

"Let food be thy medicine and medicine be thy food."

~ Hippocrates

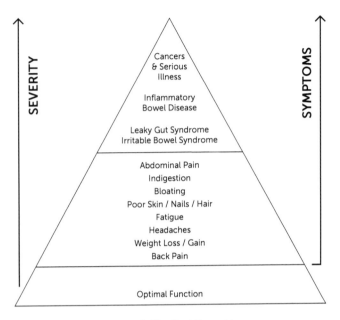

Figure 9: The Fuel Pyramid

The Fuel Pyramid is our next section of the overall model. How many times have you heard the phrase "You are what you eat"? Well, the Fuel Pyramid is about this and much more. If this only concerned what we eat then I would have called it the food pyramid, but it is not. The Fuel Pyramid is about everything that enters our body by means of eating, drinking and absorption through our skin or lungs.

As with the Framework Pyramid, there are both subjective and objective signs of aberrant function. At the bottom of the pyramid is healthy and normal function of primarily the gastrointestinal system, but also our respiratory system.

Some of the signs, symptoms and disease processes linked to factors such as diet, air pollution, and smoking are not exclusively linked to these factors. However, irritation from these factors may increase the likelihood of dysfunction leading to illness.

At the top of the pyramid would be a serious illness, including illnesses such as cancer (various forms) and ulcerative colitis. Lower, but also within the top third of the pyramid, would be conditions such as irritable bowel syndrome, leaky gut, abdominal pain, indigestion, bloating, as well as alternating constipation and diarrhoea.

The middle third would demonstrate indirect symptoms of poor function including, but not exclusively, back pain, weight loss, headaches, fatigue and poor skin and nails.

If you live in a first-world country, it is highly likely that you have the ability to control, pretty much, what you eat and drink. You can decide to smoke or not. It is harder to avoid industrial pollution, but you can live away from the 'Big Smoke' if you choose to. If, over a period of time, you ate three meals a day at a fast food outlet, smoked, drank alcohol daily and applied copious cosmetic creams to your skin daily, might that cause an undesirable effect? Let me expand on this more throughout this section.

It is Essential to Give Your Body the Right Fuel

"Sorry, there's no magic bullet. You got to eat healthy and live healthy to be healthy and look healthy. End of story."

~ Morgan Spurlock

Would you fill the fuel tank of a new Ferrari with chip fat? Of course not. But, however expensive and out of reach a new Ferrari is for the vast majority of us, it is still just a car. Money can buy you a new one. If you screw up your precious body, money cannot buy you a new one, you just have to make do and mend your current one. The lesson here is to minimise the damage as early on as possible and turn around your health.

To repeat some of our previous points, correct fuel for your body will allow you to function as you were genetically programmed to do. Economics have been at the heart of the changes we see in the diet of the modern developed world. The generation who grew up in the aftermath of the Second World War did so, in the UK and Western Europe, with ongoing food rationing. Fast food was non-existent and people drank much less alcohol than now. The only bad thing that entered their bodies that was considerably more prevalent then was cigarette smoke, and unfiltered at that!

In 1970s' USA we saw the introduction of high fructose corn syrup (HFCS). As well as being a sweetener, it was found that the introduction of HFCS acted as an effective stabiliser which led to longer shelf life for a massive range of products. HFCS is hiding inside many products and you'd have to look hard to find it. It is considered to be no coincidence that the introduction of HFCS was one of the reasons that huge weight gains were seen, especially in the USA. Its use has been clearly linked to weight gain leading to obesity, the development of Type 2 diabetes, raised blood pressure and liver damage.

This is just one example of how an imbalance in nutrients can enter our body. But I am not telling you that you need to be a monk. I will not tell you never to eat certain types of food. But we should all have our eyes opened to what it is that is entering our own body, and how that may affect our own health.

We don't eat air pollution, but we do absorb it. One of the seminars I attended whilst at the Anglo-European College of Chiropractic that has been burned into my memory was a session in the anatomy lab. Our highly-skilled tutors had been dissecting a series of cadavers for us. This was the day we were examining the respiratory system, and we were studying the lungs. Three pairs of lungs were in front of us, with one of each pair cut down through the lung to see inside. The first pair of lungs was pink with just a few specks of black visible on the outside as if someone had very lightly sprinkled some well-ground black pepper onto them. These lungs had belonged to a lady who had passed on in her eighties. She had never smoked and had always lived in the countryside, away from the big cities. They looked how I had imagined a pair of lungs to be.

The second pair was predominantly black on the outside. There were areas on the outside where there was a suggestion of the original colour but they just looked so different from the first pair we had seen. When we looked inside, though, there was a lot more pink. The dirt had made it to the extremities as this person had breathed in hard. This person had also never smoked. However, they had lived their whole life in a big conurbation and had been breathing in the smoke, dirt and pollution that is at the heart of a city. Why else are cities called 'The Big Smoke'? I was pretty shocked, especially as I had already spent four years at university in London, and breathing hard during elite sport training.

When the seminar group saw the final pair of lungs there were gasps. I was horrified. This pair was simply grim to look at. Black, not just on the outside, but pretty much throughout the interior as well. This person had been a heavy smoker their whole life, and it was amazing to me that they had lived as long as they had. How on earth did any oxygen make it into the bloodstream, and how many toxins had passed through those stunningly thin lung tissues to cross into the blood and circulate the body. How long can you live without oxygen? Not long, about 30 seconds to one minute for most people. Having seen those lungs, I could not imagine why anyone would do that to their body? I suppose the answer is deniability. Most people never get to set foot in an anatomy lab and see the damage first hand. However, all medical students do see that, so why many medical doctors smoke is a complete mystery to me!

H. Hydration

We are made of water. Well, at least two-thirds of our body is made of water. The majority of people seem to be in a mild-to-moderate state of dehydration most of the time.

During a normal 24-hour period we lose water through the natural processes of living. We get water back into our body via food and drink. Pretty obviously, if you exercise or are sweating due to heat, then you will lose a larger amount of water.

Elite sporting performers know that being even slightly dehydrated will affect their ability to perform at their best. This affects every type of activity, whether it is an endurance event or a power sprint. Becoming dehydrated leads to your blood becoming thicker. This increases resistance for the heart so your heart rate rises, and blood pressure will fall as there is less liquid within the system. Whilst your body is approximately 65% water, this percentage is much higher in the brain, which is up to 85% water. As a result, even quite minor levels of dehydration can cause you to have headaches or feel grumpy!

As well as being a chiropractor, I used to wear another hat as a rowing coach. I was the Head Coach for Headington School, Oxford, the Oxford University Women's Boat Club and the Imperial College women's team. Some of these rowing athletes made it to events such as the World Junior Rowing Championships. At these international events the physiological support was fantastic. We know that if any athlete loses even 2% of their normal water content, it will certainly start to cause a decrease in their sporting performance. Once over 3% loss, there is suddenly a much greater risk of exhaustion due to dehydration. Athletes in many sports, including rowing, spend at least two hours at a time training and can lose a much greater amount of water than 3%. This is why constant rehydration is so important.

But what about non-sporting individuals? There have been many reports suggesting that the majority of people are usually dehydrated. This can relate to both working-age people and particularly the elderly. I have known many elderly people who have almost consciously neglected to drink as this will minimise the need to get up out of their chair and go to the toilet. If they do drink in the day, it is almost exclusively tea or coffee, rather than water. Now, caffeine from tea and coffee will cause the kidneys to squeeze more water out of the body than there is in your mug of coffee in the first place!

How to recognise dehydration

A urine chart can be found easily online here (http://bit.ly/hydrationchart). I know it is not the most fun thing to do but the next time you go to the toilet have a look at the colour of your urine. We all know that the colour of urine varies. However, it should never be darker than a pale honey colour. As soon as it becomes darker, or cloudy, then your body really needs more water. Really darker yellow or orange denotes severe dehydration.

Many people rely on thirst as their indication of hydration. The problem with this is that most people will be quite severely dehydrated before they really feel thirsty. It is incredibly common to be unintentionally dehydrated, and I would go as far as to say that this is the most common situation for the vast majority of the population. A wide range of symptoms can be attributed to poor hydration levels and can include stress, headache, rising blood pressure, back pains, poor skin and certainly fatigue.

How much water should you be drinking?

One of the world's greatest experts on the effect of water on health was a medical doctor called Dr Batmanghelidj. He has an amazing story that I will not go into here, but for many years he studied the effects of water on health and he published a lot of research on the subject. He also created a calculation for working out how much water you should be drinking.

Calculate your body weight in pounds (lbs) and divide by 2. This tells you the amount of fluid ounces you need to drink.

Make this easier to understand by converting to what you know:

- Multiply by 0.0625 to tell you the quantity in pints

- Multiply by 0.0296 to calculate in litres.

It will almost certainly sound like a lot to you, probably much more than you currently drink every day.

I am a big, tall chap, standing at 6 foot 6 inches and weighing about 16 stones (224 lbs). So I need to drink about 224/2 = 112 x 0.0625 = 7 pints of water, EVERY DAY!

My patients usually look at me slightly aghast when I do the calculation for them, but if they are honest, they tell me that if they check their urine it looks dark and certainly quite yellow.

What water should you drink?

There are many schools of thought on this but I am of the opinion that if you live in a developed country then you drink your tap water. Ideally, I would pass it through a filter if you are at all uncertain about the quality of the tap water in your area, but I see no benefit in buying very expensive bottled water. If you filter the tap water, this should be able to remove any heavy metals, chemicals or pesticides that happen to be in your water.

I know some experts go as far as to say you should boil or distil all your water. I think this makes life too hard, and frankly the greater benefits will come from staying well-hydrated with clean tap water.

The final thing to do is to pop some freshly-cut and squeezed lemon or lime into your drinking water. This will help to reduce the acidity of your body's pH which helps to reduce acidosis from occurring inside you.

E. Eat

"You are what you eat." Simple. I should stop this section right here!

As you can probably tell, I believe that your amazing human body reflects how you function structurally and mentally, and of course it reflects what you are fuelling it with. The primary fuel (which I define as what enters your body via your mouth, lungs or skin) is, of course, food!

For the vast majority of our existence as humans we survived on the same hunter-gatherer diet. It is only in approximately the last 10,000-12,000 years that we learned how to use grains in food. Learning how to process hard grains, in a way that we could use easily, encouraged us to farm and develop more. This was brilliant for our ancestors, as they began to make settlements and stop roaming. They started to farm. Humans started to eat many more carbohydrates (found in grains and root vegetables), and so their percentage intake of fats and protein reduced.

If you consider the three main food groups (fat, protein and carbohydrate), it is only carbohydrate that is unessential for normal health. Intake of certain amounts of fat and protein are essential, but carbohydrate deprivation has no harmful side effects.

The way we eat, especially in the UK and USA, has evolved with our environmental evolution, population growth and agricultural technology. We clearly eat in a vastly different way now to our caveman ancestors, and even in a radically different way to 60 years ago, post the Second World War. In the UK the cost of a calorie has never been cheaper, and fast food, pre-prepared food and snacks are easily available. Is it a coincidence that there is an obesity issue in the western world? I think not!

A recent study of the common diet in the western world demonstrated many findings, but some of the stand-out points included:

- Our nutrition directly affects gene expression

- Our genes have not evolved at all since the agricultural revolution

- We eat too much omega-6 fats

- We eat too little omega-3 fats

- We eat man-made trans-fats

- We eat too many grains and grain-based foods

- We do not get enough fibre, protein, vitamin D

And finally:

- We eat too much and do not exercise enough!

What is Food?

We can break food up into different basic and well-known components. These are carbohydrate, protein, fat, vitamins, minerals and fibre. The proportion of how we take in these food types has altered socially over the years, and governments have also changed what they recommend we eat on a fairly regular basis.

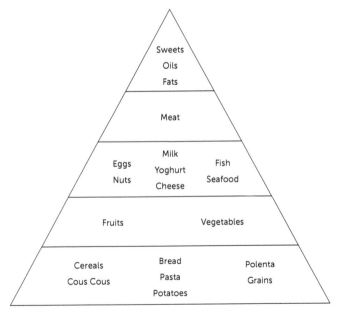

Figure 11: The 1970s' Food Pyramid

Until recently most governments recommended a food pyramid to us. This started off with the base of the pyramid, the foods we should eat the most, made up entirely of carbohydrates. The level above this was fruit and vegetables. Above this were protein and dairy products, and at the very top were fats and oils. This advice has been changed recently but I advise a different bias and will explain this later in this chapter.

Carbohydrates: can be found in various forms and can be simple or complex. Essentially all carbohydrates will be broken down, eventually, into glucose. So, the simplest carbohydrate you can ingest is sugar. These small molecules are utilised easily by your body, and they will raise the level of blood sugar faster than anything else. A complex carbohydrate means that it is a larger molecule, essentially made up of long strings of simple carbs. These large molecules need to be broken down into the simpler units to allow the body to absorb them. They will be described as 'slow release' sources of carbohydrate, but this will still be much faster than energy released from either protein or fat. Complex carbohydrates will be found in vegetables like potatoes, and in wheat (so pasta and bread are included here), rice and many other vegetables.

Just to confuse you, these carbs may also be either refined or unrefined. Refining is a production process that will inevitably cause a loss of fibre, minerals or vitamins. We know that if your diet includes too many refined carbs, risk of weight gain leading to obesity and risk of developing diabetes are both substantially increased.

Carbs are the easiest source of energy for the body to consume because they are so easy for the body to break down. An excess supply will be broken down into glycogen (which is stored inside your muscles and liver as reserve fuel – this is normal), but as soon as your glycogen supplies are full, any other carbs are then converted to fat.

The glycaemic index is a guide to how bioavailable the energy within any given food is, i.e. how fast it will cause your blood sugar levels to rise, on a scale of 1 to100. A 'Low GI' food will release slowly, while the highest 'High GI' food is sugar, and this is given a value of 100. This figure is most important in how your body will control the release of insulin. Insulin is the body's way of controlling blood sugar levels and is produced with the Islets of Langerhans in the pancreas. If you eat lots of high GI foods (imagine a massive bag of sweets), your blood sugar levels will rocket up, causing a large release of insulin. The insulin will bring the blood sugar back under control but will usually take it too far, due to a latent response, and this makes you hungry again. Keeping High GI foods out of your diet will mean there are fewer spikes in insulin release and no wild swings in your body's desire for food.

The early food pyramid used to suggest that about 50% of all your calories should come from carbohydrates. This is madness! Look around you and you will see that the vast majority of people are sedentary and overweight. Carbohydrates are not 'evil', but the fact is that most people just do not need them and will have sufficient calorific intake from fats and protein, both of which are essential to the body. We rarely get to burn the fat though, due to a massive overdose of simple carbohydrates that the body will use first because it is easy.

Protein: Proteins are made up of long chains of amino acids. Proteins are the building blocks of your body, and form the majority of structures in your body including muscles, bones, hair, collagen, enzymes, and neurotransmitters, to name just a few!

There are 20 different amino acids. Your body can make 11 of these by itself, but 9 of them are called essential amino acids as the only way we can get those is from our diet.

Some proteins are easier to access than others. The easiest to access are proteins in meat, eggs and fish. The protein that is found in some vegetables and grains is less bioavailable for the body. This makes it harder to get the correct protein levels from a vegetarian diet.

Fat: Fat is essential for life, but most people I speak to do not understand the mechanisms involved and think of all fat as bad, especially as they check their waistband measurement! Don't get me wrong – there are some types of fat which are very bad for you as well as some fat that is essential for life.

What are the bad fats? The worst of all are trans fatty acids, otherwise known as trans fats. These are artificial, i.e. not found naturally and are man-made. They were designed by food scientists to increase the shelf life of many baked goods, and so are now found in the majority of commercially prepared food which is made with partially hydrogenated vegetable oil.

Trans fats (also known as hydrogenated or partially hydrogenated fats on food labels) will increase the levels of the 'bad' cholesterol in your blood and, simultaneously, lower the levels of the essential 'good' cholesterol. Trans fats have also been linked to raising your risk of developing Type 2 diabetes and heart disease.

Why are trans fats so bad for you?

Approximately 80% of the cell wall of every cell in your body is made of fat, while the remaining 20% is made of protein. The protein element of the cell wall makes shape-specific receptor sites which are how cell function is controlled via hormones or neurotransmitters. These protein receptor sites are very sensitive to being distorted, and if this happens their ability to function is affected.

The fat that forms the cell wall of every cell in your body is derived from what you eat. So literally, "You are what you eat". Trans fats are very long, and extremely stiff. As such, when they become integrated into new cell walls they stiffen, and distort the cell wall. One of the most sensitive of these receptor sites is the insulin receptor. If the body cannot respond normally to insulin release, the body initially responds by increasing insulin production, to swamp the receptor sites. However, if this fails, then you lose correct function allowing you to balance blood sugar levels, i.e. you develop Type 2 diabetes.

Due to their size trans fats are harder for your body to get rid of, so it is known that they start to accumulate within you, and their adverse effect begin to accumulate.

What else do we know about trans fats?

- Trans fats adversely affect the correct ratio of (good) high density lipoprotein cholesterol and (bad) low density lipoprotein, so this will increase your chance of heart disease or stroke.

- Trans fats will pass across a placenta to a mother's unborn child.

- Trans fats reduce your body's ability to absorb Vitamin K, which is required for good bone health.

- Trials have shown that there may be a link between trans fats and increased risk of developing prostate cancer.

This is not an exhaustive list of all the dangers of trans fats but demonstrates a wide range of the many dangers linked to this artificial fat type.

The good news is that your body is slowly replacing and regenerating every day. It is estimated that your body creates about 300 billion new cells every day. If you eliminate these trans fats from your diet, you will, over time, replace these unhealthy fats and the function of new cells will be normal. However, you will be in the minority of people. Most people will keep on eating their diet that is rich in trans fats, so their health will deteriorate as the percentage of this fat type in their body increases.

Denmark became the first country in the world to introduce laws strictly regulating the sale of many foods containing trans fats in March 2003. Over a decade has passed since then, and health statistics from Denmark show that deaths due to cardiovascular disease have dropped very significantly. In the early years of the ban, deaths due to cardiovascular disease lowered by 4%. Denmark then tightened its anti-smoking laws, and the levels of death due to cardiovascular disease took an even greater jump in the right direction. Are you going to head out now for a burger and fries?

Essential fatty acids

One of my core beliefs as a chiropractor is that I can improve nervous system function by both improving the biomechanics of the spine, by removing vertebral restrictions (subluxation), and by integrating brain and body function. However, I also know that normal neurological function requires a specific ratio in the blood between omega-6 and omega-3 fatty acids.

Omega-3 and omega-6 are both essential fatty acids and are both polyunsaturated fatty acids (PUFA). Whereas the 'evil' trans fats are extremely long and very stiff, these fatty acids can bend. The numbers, 3 and 6, relate to the numbers of double bonds in the chain and these fat molecules can bend and twist at these points. This is the simple reason why animal fat will solidify at room temperature, whereas a bottle of cod liver oil can sit in the fridge and will still be liquid. After all, the poor cod would be in trouble swimming around in the Arctic if what little fat it had was frozen!

We think that our hunter-gatherer ancestors ate a diet that was roughly 1:1 in a ratio of omega 6:omega 3. Estimates now suggest that many of us now consume a ratio of about

25:1, and that this is due to a lack of omega 3 in our diet. This should be scary in lots of ways, especially as up to 40% of the fatty acids found in the cell walls in the brain are omega 3. If the ratio of omega 6:omega 3 is too far off from the designed one, then abnormal function will occur and your body will not maintain homeostasis. This will inevitably lead to illness and disease.

This great change in the correct ratio of these essential fatty acids has occurred particularly in the last 150 years or so, as we have consumed huge amounts of vegetable oils, and so omega-6 levels have been very high. At the same time natural levels of omega-3 oils have dropped, as farming methods have become more forced.

Omega-3 oils are found in two forms that have very complex names. I will refer to them by their shortened names, EPA and DHA. It is the DHA levels in particular that are so important for brain development and function, anti-ageing (lack of this affects cognitive function and memory), and also pre-natal brain development.

Omega-3 deficiency has been linked, by research, to a huge variety of conditions including depression, cancer, heart disease, arthritis, allergies, violent behaviour and weight gain. The majority of us are deficient in omega-3 and some will be extremely deficient. There is also a link between socio-economic groups and prevalence of deficiency. This is because those who are struggling to feed their families, such as the 'working poor', simply cannot afford the food types that are rich in omega-3, and the food that they can afford is usually both low in fatty acids and high in those trans fats. A double whammy! Studies of prison inmates have also shown that offenders of violent crime have a very high ratio of omega-6:omega-3. But you will struggle to get enough omega-3 fatty acids into your body even with taking a look at your diet. Our ancestors got much more from their diets of green leaves, fish and meat than we can get from mass produced crops. Sadly, our seas are now full of pollution, and eating fresh fish too often may actually lead to a dangerous consumption of heavy metals and PCP's, which is very sad but true. I recommend taking a high quality omega-3 supplement fish oil that has been extracted to a pharmaceutical grade, i.e. it has been distilled from the wild fish and even the tiniest trace amounts of these chemicals have been removed. I will discuss these vital supplements further in the Life Supplements section of this chapter.

Primal Eating – aka 'Eat Like your Ancestors'

What is Primal Eating?

I have described many of the basics of primal eating at various points in this section of the book. Human beings ate a very similar diet for several hundreds of thousands of years during prehistoric times while we lived exclusively as hunter-gatherers. Approximately 12,000-15,000 years ago came the agricultural revolution and we learned how to farm due to gaining knowledge of how to process hard grains for food.

One of the earliest civilisations to develop the farming of cereal crops was the Egyptians. Whilst they have left a few amazing relics of their building prowess, there are few signs of their farming. However, they did like to mummify their nearest and dearest, and this has allowed modern-day archaeological pathologists to assess their health, lives and causes of death. We know that the Egyptians ate a high carbohydrate and low fat diet, consisting of bread and other cereals, fresh fruit and vegetables, some fish and fowl but hardly any red meat. This is what modern day nutritionists have been recommending to us for many years, so surely the ancient Egyptians were tremendously healthy? Sadly, they were not!

In his book *Protein Power*, Dr Michael Eades describes how the mummified remains of many ancient Egyptians demonstrate a very different outcome. It appears that they suffered from obesity, severe tooth decay (despite the lack of refined sugars in their diet), and very clear, and widespread, arterial disease. Does this sound like the typical body type, and dis-ease, that is prevalent in western societies to this present day? I think so, and it is a great shame that this has not been recognised widely. As I write this book, the UK government has just increased its recommendations from eating 5 portions of fresh fruit or vegetables every day to 10 portions. Is this the correct number, or should it be more? The government has indicated that it knew that we should be eating at least 10 portions at the time of the previous recommendation, but the general public would not 'swallow' such claims at the time! Recently the recommended 'food pyramid' has also changed to move fruit and vegetables to the base of the pyramid, and carbohydrate is now one step up reflecting that grains and cereals should NOT be the foundation of our diets. Frankly, they should only complement our diet, not be a pillar of it.

In the USA in the 1970s the government recommended that people reduced their fat intake significantly, after the work of one man linked fat to heart disease. It was at this point that it was recommended to increase carbohydrate levels. Prior to this point, less than 20% of either males or females had been obese in the USA. Since that time, obesity levels have escalated rapidly, and continue to rise. Currently over a third of the US adult population is obese, leading to tremendous health and social issues throughout the country.

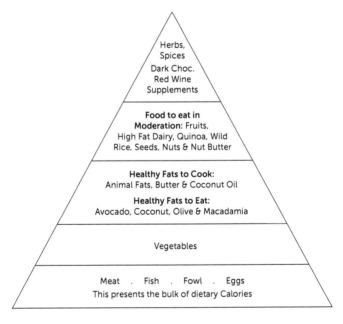

Figure 12: The Primal Food Pyramid

Primal Eating takes us back to the basics and natural food. Don't panic, as this can still be super yummy! At this stage let me make this really simple. In an ideal world the ideal primal eating pattern would mean:

- No processed foods

- No sugar and other refined carbohydrates

- No grains

- No dairy *

- No alcohol **

- Eat like a wolf, not like a podgy bear – i.e. do not overeat!

- Avoid like the plague – high fructose corn syrup, trans fats, monosodium glutamate, aspartame

- Eat lots of fresh vegetables – raw, steamed or lightly cooked

- Fish, meat – grass-fed meat

* Regarding dairy, I think it OK to have a little splash of full-fat milk in your coffee or a little cheese in your omelette, but most people simply consume far too much. So, high-fat dairy products, in moderation, are fine. Likewise, Kefir (a fermented form of milk) has amazing health benefits for you.

** Stay away from beer (it is made from grain) and enjoy a nice glass of red wine instead. Let's be reasonable though. Am I teetotal? No, I have to admit a loving for a gorgeously deep red wine. Red wine has lots of anti-oxidants in it, but don't go crazy!

Life is a balance. Most people have the balance totally out of whack. If you can follow the guidelines the majority of the time, that would benefit you greatly, so find what you can sustain and stick to it.

A: Absorbed by your body

While the most prevalent way that chemicals enter our bodies is by way of our mouths, a huge amount gets into us either through our lungs or skin. If you live, or work, in a city, you will be exposed to many more pollutants from vehicle traffic than if you live in the countryside. Do you smoke, or does your partner? Do you apply liberal quantities of makeup, sun cream or topical painkilling cream? What do we know about some of these major topics?

Where you live affects your health?

There is a large, and growing, amount of research on the effects of pollution, and as we see this documented we start to put another piece of the health jigsaw in place, rather than just assuming something is true. It has only very recently been demonstrated that living in close proximity to a major road can increase your risk of developing dementia. It was found that about 10% of deaths due to dementia were directly linked to air pollution, and that when you live further away from the busiest roads, your risk factors diminish accordingly. I find it staggering that dementia is now the leading cause of death in the United Kingdom in both men and women, and that the number of deaths due to dementia, including of course Alzheimer's Disease, is rising rapidly year on year. Why now? What is the true underlying cause of this horrendous spectrum of conditions?

Other than the various forms of dementia, ongoing exposure to elevated levels of air pollution can lead to inflammation, breathing issues, and even to serious heart disease and cancers.

Smoking was only ever 'cool' for the Marlboro Man!

Other than because of the huge tax revenues it brings in, I am amazed that smoking is still legal in developed countries. My mind was completely blown about 12 years ago when my wife, Laura, and I arrived at the John Radcliffe Hospital in Oxford for the imminent arrival of our first child. Every time I entered or left the maternity department there was always a small group of heavily pregnant ladies smoking outside the entrance! Simply unbelievable! After seeing this, I look out for similar sightings whenever I go past a hospital. Smokers huddle outside the hospital entrances, and this seems to be considered normal.

I have already described my experience of looking at several pairs of dissected human lungs. This was genuinely shocking to me as we compared smokers with non-smokers and city dwellers with those who had lived in the countryside. I think I have smoked a maximum of two dozen cigarettes in my life, between the ages of 17 and 20, so like most people I have tried them, but seeing those lungs made me extremely happy that I had not taken up this habit.

Smoking is declining in popularity, but about 7 to 8 million people still smoke in the UK, and smoking is, without doubt, the leading cause of premature death! Heart disease, stroke, many forms of cancer and severe lung disease are the primary killers. I will not describe the mechanics of the various disease processes that smoking causes as this can be found elsewhere. However, as well as these killer diseases there is a huge range of other processes that also affect any smoker.

If you smoke, you will age faster. Smoking alters your skin, hair and teeth. If you smoke, the blood supply to the skin decreases, causing a lack of oxygen to the skin and this will damage both collagen and elastin. This makes your skin saggy and loose. If you are a smoker, you are much more likely to suffer from sight loss, develop gum disease and have grotty bad breath.

On a structural (framework) front, smokers are much more likely to lose bone strength, and this may lead on to osteoporosis. This occurs as the effect of the toxins, especially nicotine and huge quantities of free radicals, within the smoke inhibit the function of the osteoblasts, or bone creating cells. The osteoblasts actually get killed, and if the smoking continues they cannot be replaced fast enough!

Also, remember when I discussed stress and hormone production. The primary stress hormone is cortisol. Smoking causes an increase in cortisol levels (ironic that people smoke because they are stressed and yet the very action of smoking will increase cortisol release), and one action of cortisol is to cause bone breakdown.

For many years, and indeed while I was growing up, the iconic 'Marlboro Man' summed up everything that was 'cool' about smoking and what it 'did for you'. Well, there is nothing cool about smoking, especially in the way it harms children if you smoke in the house or in the car. The Marlboro Man must have the final word on the subject of smoking though. At least four of these advertising icons have died from smoking related disease. Let's move on.

What do you absorb through your skin?

We put a lot onto our skin and think nothing of it, often imagining that it is impermeable. But how can it be impermeable when we stick nicotine or hormone replacement therapy patches to the skin and expect that this will be absorbed correctly? Then think about the tens of thousands of litres of lotions we apply every year. Whether this is sun cream, body cream, shampoo, make-up or perfumes, do we know what is in them and could they be harmful?

The good news is that the vast majority of chemical compounds cannot penetrate all layers of the skin and get into the bloodstream. Most compounds are just too large to be absorbed, and others often need an associated chemical to help the process of penetration. Also, it is true that absorption into the body does not necessarily equate to being harmful. The safety of any chemical is related to the amount that is both absorbed and accumulated over time.

So why is it that studies of the umbilical cords of babies have shown a vast number of toxins within them? The truth is that some chemicals do make it into the body when ideally they should not be getting in. Some make it through hair follicles or sweat ducts and from there get to either the bloodstream or lymphatic system.

Skincare and other cosmetics can even be taken in orally. Lead is sometimes found in lipsticks for example. If a lady reapplies her lipstick several times every day, then dangerous amounts of toxin could be ingested.

Our skin is not the totally impregnable barrier that we often think it is. There are other things that we sometimes block out with chemical barriers that we actually need. The classic case here is Vitamin D deprivation. I will talk much more about Vitamin D in a later part of this chapter on Life Supplements, but I find it very scary that there are a growing number of reports of rickets (due to Vitamin D deficiency) in the UK every year.

Rickets affects young children as their bones are developing, growing and strengthening. Parents have become terrified of the dangers of skin cancer. As a result of this the use of high factor sun creams has increased. However, if you are completely covered up whenever playing outside, then there is little chance you will be exposed to sufficient direct sunlight. Compound the sunscreen use with more playing on computers, increased TV and a nutritionally poor diet, and we see this, previously eradicated, disease making a comeback. I regularly recommend simple bloodspot tests to my patients to check their Vitamin D levels if there is a chance that it could be low. Once these levels drop, the only way to get the levels up again in a time efficient way is by use of supplements.

I recommend looking at what is in the products that you regularly apply to yourself. Is there a long list of weird-looking names in the ingredients? Are you spraying aluminium antiperspirants into your armpits? Where possible I recommend using natural products, or simply minimising the use of some of these potions and lotions.

L: Life supplements

'Do I need to take supplements?' 'Are they just a waste of money?' 'I eat a great diet so do I really need to take these?'

These are just some of the many questions that get fired at me on a regular basis in my clinic. Now while I have been banging on about how our hunter-gatherer ancestors lived, it is quite clear that none of them ever took supplements. However, they did not need to do this. They ate a very nutritionally rich diet of 100% organic food. They drank clean spring water, were never exposed to pollution or pesticides, ate no processed foods and exercised loads!

Our industrialised farming techniques mean that the soil has lost much of its natural nutrients. The meat we produce has virtually zero healthy fatty acids any more and the seas are full of pollutants. Our environment has developed very fast and there are only a handful of hunter-gatherers left now, and none of them are in the UK or USA!

It has become essential for us to use a few 'Life Supplements' to ensure that we meet our ideal nutritional intake.

Omega-3 fish oils

Recent research from Harvard University pronounced that deficiency of omega-3 fatty acids was one on the top 10 causes of death in the USA. Two things stand out to me here:

1. If there were many deaths attributable to lack of omega-3 fatty acids, then how many people were seriously or moderately ill through an omega-3

deficiency less severe than that suffered by the fatalities?

2. Deficiency of omega-3 is totally preventable if appropriate supplements are given. The sad thing, though, is that they may be unaffordable to many people.

The many benefits of fish oils include, but are not limited to:

1. ADHD: As Attention Deficit Hyperactivity Disorder has become a more prevalent problem, an increase in omega-3 has been shown to improve behaviour and school performance.

2. Alzheimer's disease: These fish oils may have a benefit in the prevention of onset of Alzheimer's and have certainly shown a slowing of disease development, and brain shrinking is minimised with its use.

3. Arthritis: A very exciting study has shown a far greater benefit in the use of omega-3 supplementation for the benefit of rheumatoid arthritis than with any other form of therapy. As regards osteoarthritis (degenerative joint disease), studies have shown that omega-3 outperformed ibuprofen for the benefit of pain relief.

4. Cancer: There have been a number of studies now demonstrating a reduction in, and treatment benefit for, many forms of cancer, particularly breast cancer. As well as being beneficial on its own, there is an even greater benefit in combining omega-3

supplementation with some anti-cancer medication.

5. Heart disease: I discussed this earlier when talking diet and primal eating. Eating a high fat, low carbohydrate diet that is rich in omega-3 fatty acids is very beneficial for your heart.

6. Diabetes: Amongst other studies there are amazing benefits for diabetics in preventing damage to the retinas in their eyes with sufficient omega-3 in their diet.

7. Skin and hair: The benefits are again due to reduced inflammation, and can benefit conditions including eczema, psoriasis and dandruff.

8. Depression: Clinical supplementation in depressive adolescents showed a huge benefit and improvements in mood and a lifting of the symptoms of depression.

Whilst the best way to get your omega-3 fish oils would be to enjoy some wild cold water fish, such as salmon or sardines, the sad truth is that these fish have nasty levels of heavy metals and pesticides such as PCP in them. I recommend using a high quality supplement of at least 1000 milligrams per day for the average-sized person, but you may take more if you are larger or if you are demonstrating any signs or symptoms of deficiency. These levels also depend on the rest of your diet. If you are still taking in trans fats, for example, then this must be addressed and reduced, and raise the levels of the healthy fish oils.

Omega-3 fish oils really are one of the most important nutrients you could take, both for yourself and every member of your family, and for life! You need the correct balance of omega-3 to ensure good health and balance your modern diet. This entire book is about proactive health that will create lasting change, so please add omega-3 fish oils to your diet.

Vitamin D

Vitamin D is actually not a nutritional compound, but is a hormone. The most common way your body produces Vitamin D is within your cells using the power of sunlight. The body's need for vitamin D is essential, and is involved with many systems in the body especially muscle function, bone growth (the worst cases of vitamin D deficiency leading to rickets in young children) and the inflammatory process. There are also strong links to vitamin D being very important in cancer prevention. What can be very scary is that in many cases someone can become very seriously deficient in vitamin D and still be asymptomatic.

I had a patient who had been suffering ongoing muscular, and bone, aches and pains. It was only when his medical doctor carried out a full series of blood tests, and vitamin D levels were included, that his levels were discovered as being very low. Since then I offer bloodspot tests for this at the clinic as vitamin D deficiency is much more common that many people think.

Some of the possible symptoms that may be linked to low levels of vitamin D may include: ongoing aches and pains, pain in the joints, headache, muscle cramp, fatigue, weakness, depressed immunity leading to regular colds and poor sleep quality.

The best source of getting your regular vitamin D is from the sun. You really need to be getting about 15 minutes every day onto your arms and legs. This may be tricky if you are commuting to work every day and are indoors, and it may be cold, wet and windy at the weekends. If you have dark skin, you must be outside in the sun even more. So someone whose body has evolved to live near the equator will struggle for vitamin D if they are living nearer to one of the Poles, and will be at greater risk of illness caused by a low level of vitamin D. Whilst not the primary source, you can get vitamin D from some food sources, especially cod liver oil and wild salmon.

Probiotics:

Do you know how your small and large intestine work? Or is it another area of your body that you take for granted a little bit? As food, of various sources, enters the body and makes its way into the digestive tract, the gut has a huge role in protecting us, as well as digesting the food. Many health problems, including chronic fatigue, joint pain, psoriasis and some thyroid problems, can all start in the gut.

So, what are probiotics? The World Health Organization's definition is: "Live organisms which when administered in adequate amounts confer a health benefit on the host". If you look at how the body develops through the study of embryology, you see that the gut, all the way from your mouth to your anus, is considered to be the outside world to your body. Within the gut you are the hosts to a massive amount of bacteria. Estimates suggest that there are more than 10 times more bacteria living within your digestive tract than there are cells in your body!

The vast majority of people need to have their levels of probiotic bacteria boosted and supported. This is due to the constant barrage the gut is under from our modern diet. The balance within the gut is challenged by unhealthy bacteria, fungal infections, viruses and even microbial parasites. This barrage, as I call it, is due to a massive overload of sugar, other refined carbohydrates, alcohol and grains, and at the same time we are low in natural fibre from fruit and vegetables. We also know how powerful an effect on gut function many prescription medicines can be. Even over the counter medicines can often alter your bowel function noticeably.

How about antibiotics? You have heard all the reports about how commonly prescribed these 'wonder drugs' are. Antibiotics will have a very powerful, and adverse, effect on bowel function. You don't need to eat or drink anything, though, to affect the bowels. I described earlier the many effects of stress on the body. Stress very quickly changes blood flow and neural response to the intestines, and yet people can be in a stressed state for months or even years! For these reasons, and many more, addressing the health of your gastro-intestinal tract (from top to bottom!) needs to be a priority.

The deficiency of healthy gut bacteria commonly occurs at birth. Babies develop their gut bacteria from their mother. This process is designed to start during a normal vaginal birth, and then almost immediately from their mother's breast milk. But many children are now delivered by Caesarean section, so they miss out there, and an ever-increasing number are never breast fed, so they miss out not just on these healthy bacteria but also they do not receive mum's immune system through her breast milk. If we start life like this, and we know that the average person's diet is extremely deficient in healthy probiotic bacteria, it is unlikely that a normal balance of gut bacteria will develop.

Common symptoms associated with low levels of healthy probiotic bacteria can include irregular digestion (indigestion or feeling very bloated), halitosis (bad breath), candida and skin issues (including acne and eczema).

A healthy balance of probiotics in your gut could allow you to enjoy:

- More regular digestive function

- Better immune system

- Improved eczema and psoriasis

- Reducing risk of immuno-inflammatory disease (including ulcerative colitis and diabetes)

- Fewer colds

- Increased energy

One of the best ways to boost your probiotic bacteria is with some really healthy foods including:

1. Kefir: This is essentially fermented milk, which doesn't make it sound too appealing. Kefir is made from milk and fermented kefir grains. The fermentation process also breaks down the lactose, making this a fabulous boost for those who are lactose intolerant.

   Kefir has been shown to provide massive benefits to your health. Consuming fermented foods can reduce the number of cancerous cells in the body. Kefir is also brilliant for bone health. The healthy bacteria within the kefir (probiotics) make you more efficient at absorbing key nutrients for bone health, nutrients such as calcium, magnesium and vitamin D.

   Whilst most commonly kefir is made with milk, it is also possible to make it using coconut milk, which means it will be 100% dairy free and will still give you all the probiotic benefits, as well as all the benefits of fantastic coconut milk, especially its really high levels of potassium and electrolytes.

   You can make either form of kefir at home. All you have to do is buy a culture starter kit, and you can have your first batch of fresh, homemade kefir in a matter of days.

2. Sauerkraut: I remember when I was growing up and laughing when I heard the word 'sauerkraut' because it just sounded funny, and I didn't know (or care) what it actually was. When someone told me that it was a form of fermented cabbage, I probably

pulled the worst face you can imagine (although if I tell this to one of my young children, they will still pull the same face even though they eat it). However, sauerkraut has been an extremely popular food through the centre of Europe for centuries. Fermentation was one of the most successful methods of preserving food before we had electricity, refrigerators or inert gas packing methods!

As with kefir, there is a wide-ranging list of benefits of fermented food that have been well researched, including improvements to a range of digestive disorders, mood problems (such as depression), diabetes, food allergies and even asthma!

It is possible to find easy recipes for sauerkraut if you search the ubiquitous Google.

3. Kimchi: Kimchi is the national dish of Korea. It is both yummy and very good for you. It has been eaten by Koreans for many hundreds of years, and mostly because it lasted and tasted great, rather than for its health benefits. As with the other two fermented foods I am concentrating on here, the fermentation process itself creates the healthy bacteria. These healthy bacteria, once they have established themselves in your gut, will suppress the action of any harmful bacteria and will effectively clean inside your intestine. This will benefit similar conditions to all those already mentioned.

There are plenty of other very healthy foods that you could consume as well. Lots of people ask me about probiotic yoghurts. These have become very popular and most do contain some probiotic bacteria. However, my 'gut' feel for these yoghurts is that they are marketed with quite a large premium on them due to their health-giving properties. They certainly won't do you any harm, and if you enjoy them, then eating them is better for you than not.

Over the last few years I have had more and more people telling me about their use of apple cider vinegar for a range of conditions. As they told me, I needed to find out more and did my research. It is a fantastic remedy with many possible uses. As with many healthy natural products, there has recently been a much greater amount of research into its possible benefits. Some of the benefits include an ability to lower your blood pressure, help with controlling acid reflux and a benefit to diabetes.

The research on the effects of apple cider vinegar on blood pressure was conducted in 2009, and followed a sample group over a 12-week trial. This resulted in the vinegar-taking group seeing a significant reduction in blood pressure readings.

Apple cider vinegar is another naturally fermented product. As a result of this process it produces both acetic acid and probiotic bacteria. Unlike the previously mentioned foods, the probiotics are less important here compared to the acetic acid that can help to control the acid-alkali balance in the body.

Other probiotic, healthy, fermented foods include Japanese miso and eastern European kvass.

What about probiotic supplements?

So, having mentioned many of the natural food types that can boost your gut's probiotic bacteria, what about supplements? Are they necessary? The simple answer is that if your overall diet is not rich enough in natural probiotic bacteria then you need to boost this with more. The bacteria within capsule supplements are very similar strains to those found occurring naturally in the gut, but these have been grown specifically for this use.

It is my belief that the vast majority of the population would benefit from actively increasing their probiotic bacteria in the gut. And this applies to all age groups, especially the young, elderly and expecting mothers.

The main thing you have to be careful about when purchasing probiotics capsules is that many of these supplements are destroyed by the acid in your stomach before they have a chance to reach the intestine and start to colonise the gut. So, what do you need to check for on the packaging?

- High levels of probiotic bacteria: Each capsule should contain anywhere from 15-100 billion bacteria.

- Bacteria type: Look for certain bacteria types that have a good chance of surviving into the gut, such as Lactobacillus Acidophilus, Bifidobacteria Lactis, Lactobacillus Salivarius and Lactobacillus Plantarum.

- Has it been chilled? These supplements need to be kept in the cold to minimise the loss of bacteria. How have they been stored?

- Expiry: How long is left on their 'Best Before' date? These are living things. If the expiry date is soon then they have been bottled up for a long time.

Magnesium

Magnesium is, in my opinion, the most important mineral for your body. It has a very important series of functions in your body and is crucial to the regulation of other minerals including calcium, potassium and sodium. So, how is it that magnesium deficiency is now very prevalent? There are several key reasons why. Firstly, as we know, most of our agricultural farming land has been industrially farmed since World War Two. As such, many key minerals have been leached away and as a result the quantity of minerals in resulting crops has decreased. Secondly, for a variety of reasons we have become less adept at actually absorbing what minerals are present in food. It is really hard to put a number on the proportion of people who are magnesium deficient, but it may be as high as 80% of the population.

What are some of the key symptoms of magnesium deficiency?

1. Cramp: Cramping of the muscles, especially the calf muscles, is the most common symptom. This is because both flexing and contracting muscles are active processes. This means it takes energy and

cellular action to facilitate. As you contract a muscle, calcium enters each muscle cell, and as it does so, magnesium exits. This system should work in reverse to relax. However, as we have loads of calcium (in our bones), it is unlikely to get deficient in this, whereas a deficiency in magnesium happens easily and we struggle to then replace it. This is best helped by magnesium supplements.

2. High Blood Pressure: It has been shown that a diet that is rich in magnesium can reduce your risk of stroke significantly. High Blood Pressure is linked to the majority of strokes occurring.

3. Osteoporosis: Most of the magnesium that is normally in your body is found in your bones. Increasing the magnesium levels, and vitamin D as well, can slow down the progression of osteoporosis.

4. Diabetes: Magnesium plays a very important role in the metabolism of sugar. A magnesium-rich diet can lower the risk of developing Type 2 diabetes by around 15%!

There are plenty of other symptoms and actions of magnesium, including raising your energy levels, reducing your anxiety, helping your digestion and also helping to prevent migraines.

'How much extra magnesium do I need, and where can I get it from?' This is a vital question and especially for this mineral. This is because taking too much extra magnesium can cause you to suffer diarrhoea. So keep to within the recommended amounts and avoid more than 400 milligrams per day.

Magnesium is found in lots of really green leafed vegetables, spinach being the richest (now you know why Popeye loved it!). It is also found in good quantities in black beans, avocados, almonds and cashew nuts, bananas, broccoli and even good old potatoes.

Antioxidants

Lots of people I speak to are uncertain what antioxidants are and whether they are important or not. An antioxidant is simply something that inhibits the process of oxidation. Just by living and with the daily biochemical reactions occurring in the body, our cells will produce 'free radicals'. Some free radicals can be very useful and are made by the liver to help break down certain toxins. However, if the natural ratio of antioxidants to free radicals inside you becomes skewed, so that there are too few antioxidants, then the excess free radicals can cause quite a lot of damage.

Some of the effects of excess free radicals may cause your body to age faster. This can affect all tissue types in the body, especially your skin, joints, brain and heart. Free radicals can damage the DNA within every cell, along with cell membranes and the enzymes that pass between cells.

There are some 'superfoods' that have become high-profile 'fashion foods' because of their antioxidant levels. These include goji berries, blueberries, pecan nuts and kidney beans. However, you can also benefit from other great foods such as tomatoes, carrots, broccoli, kale and even... red wine!

Whilst I do not think you have to go crazy and force yourself to search out and eat tons of goji berries, I do think that this emphasises the benefit of lots of raw, or steamed, fruits, salads and vegetables in your diet. As I have said before, it is now very well known how deficient the most commonly eaten diet in the UK or USA is in these healthy foods, and yet they are so simple to include in your day-to-day life.

Summary

Eating food that is rich in vitamins may protect your cells, and especially the chromosomal telomeres, from the damage of oxidation. Highly antioxidant foods may slow the rate of ageing and will also play a role in preventing cellular damage. Even after reading the advice in this chapter, if you feel that your diet may continue to be insufficient, then a study has demonstrated that taking a regular multivitamin can slightly increase telomere length. And as I continue to repeat, chromosomal telomere length is a direct measure of ageing, and of your health.

So, **H.E.A.L. Yourself From The Inside Out!**

6

The Feel Pyramid –
F.E.E.L. Alive!

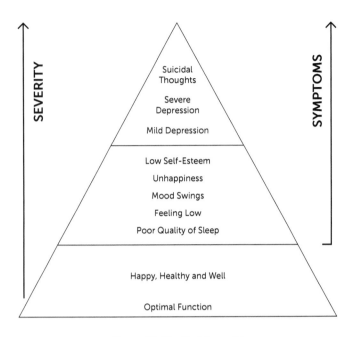

Figure 13: The Feel Pyramid

"The mind can go either direction under stress — toward positive or toward negative: on or off. Think of it as a spectrum whose extremes are unconsciousness at the negative end and hyperconsciousness at the positive end. The way the mind will lean under stress is strongly influenced by training."

~ Frank Herbert, Dune

An Introduction to F.E.E.L.

"F.E.E.L. Alive!"

- **F. is for FOCUS:** Can you recognise if you are, or someone else is feeling down or becoming depressed? How can you improve your mood and explore the mind/body link?

- **E. is for ENVIRONMENTAL:** How do your surroundings, relationships, upbringing, society pressures and traumatic events affect your mental health?

- **E. is for ENERGY:** The mind is one of the biggest contributors of energy levels for both mental and physical energy. What can you do to increase your energy?

- **L. is for LOVE:** We need to be able to love ourselves to be happy. As Mahatma Gandhi said: "Where there is love there is life."

What Are The Effects Of Chiropractic Adjustments On The Mind?

Chiropractic adjustments can increase positive body thoughts and decrease negative body thoughts. The mind/ body link works in both directions.

The Feel Pyramid is our next section of the overall model. I have always felt, known and observed in practice that physical stress and mental stress are absolutely entwined. If I am asked to play charades at Christmas, or I am trying to mime something, I am pretty rubbish. However, I think that all of us can mime stress very well. This is an emotion that most people, when asked, will demonstrate in the same way. You would clench your teeth, make your hands into fists, shrug your shoulders and maybe stick your chin out. You would also recognise this instantly, because we subconsciously read these signals every single day from people all around us.

The Feel Pyramid relates not just to mental stress, but to mental health as well. Imagine you are a millionaire playboy, living on an amazing yacht in Monaco. You have everything you could imagine but you suffer ongoing, chronic pain. Are you happy? No chance. If this persists, you would become depressed which can also affect your overall health. On the other hand, you may be an Olympian at the absolute peak of physical function. But there's a problem: something is causing you anxiety or anguish and worry. However hard you have trained, do you think you will be able to perform at your physical best? I think it is highly unlikely.

As with the other pyramids, there are both subjective and objective signs of aberrant function. At the bottom of the pyramid is healthy and normal function, i.e. optimal mental health. You could say someone here would feel happy, healthy and well.

At the top of the pyramid would be serious illness. At the very peak of the pyramid would be the very scary possibility of suicidal thoughts, irrational behaviour and very severe depression. The mildest of the subjective symptoms would be mild depression.

The middle third of the pyramid would demonstrate the precursors to a more severe problem. These might include mood swings, feeling a bit low, trouble sleeping and a general feeling of unhappiness.

The Feel Pyramid clearly demonstrates a significant overlap with the entire chapter on Stress, and the physiological effects that stress can cause on the body.

It is essential for your overall health to have great mental health

The UK mental health charity, Mind, estimates that 1 in every 4 people in the UK will experience a mental health problem every year! These problems can include disorders such as depression, anxiety, panic attacks, OCD and eating disorders.

As regards the most serious of these issues, it is thought that these can be better estimated over the course of someone's lifetime. Approximately 15-20 in every 100 people may suffer from suicidal thoughts! This is much more prevalent even than those who will self-harm. Whilst a much smaller number actually follow through with these terrible thoughts, there are about 4,000 suicides in the UK every year.

Another crushing illness is dementia. This crippling mental illness is becoming ever more prevalent, and we don't know why this is. There are currently about 850,000 people suffering from Alzheimer's disease and this is forecast to increase to over one million within the next 10 years, and to double in the following 25 years.

There is now an overload in demand for the provision of mental health services in the UK, and there is a similar pattern throughout the western world. What is it that has caused this great increase in dementia rates? Part of the answer is that dementia rates do increase with age, and there is an ever-increasing number of elderly people, so some increase in dementia sufferers will be inevitable. But there is also an increase in the number of younger dementia sufferers.

The connection between the mind and the body is called psychoneurophysiology, and is vital for a natural approach to healing and wellness. Psychoneurophysiology essentially examines the way that your mind and nervous system work together. There are messages moving from the brain to the body, and vice versa, from the body to the brain. Studies have clearly shown that irritated spinal function will send nociceptive (pain giving) signals to the brain whilst simultaneously decreasing healthy proprioceptive (movement) signals. At the same time, if brain function is irritated, this will cause dysfunction to the body.

This is something that can be affected when using the Neurological Integration System (NIS). As I have mentioned, a physical stress, such as a spinal subluxation, will send pain signals that cause a stress reaction within the amygdala, which is the stress and fear centre within the brain. So, we know that pain felt by the body is sent as messages to the brain and that the brain reacts to these in the same way as a stressful thought. Likewise, normal body movement sends this as positive feedback to the brain. Your brain would respond to this as healthy, normal, positive stimulus, i.e. the same as a happy thought.

F: Focus

What do I mean by FOCUS? The ability to focus, and identify, one's thoughts, to maintain attention and recognise one's mood.

Recognise if you're down (or someone you love is down)

'Feeling down' is very common. If this is something that is only occasional for you, then it is nothing to worry about. We are not robots, living in a linear state of being. If you feel exhilarated one moment, then there is every chance that another scenario will leave you feeling anything but exhilarated! However, I believe that we should be more open about our moods and be better able to share how we feel. Men are clearly worse at this and often keep their thoughts to themselves. It is still quite a taboo subject to talk about depression, let alone other forms of mental health challenges.

Here are some of the common signs of 'feeling down':

- Becoming withdrawn

- Needing more stimulant – commonly alcohol and caffeine

- No enthusiasm for life, work or family

- Mood swings – especially if this pattern has changed recently

- Becoming quick to anger

- Loss of direction and uncertainty

- Withdrawing from socialising and preferring one's own company

- Sleeping issues – too much or too little, also waking unrefreshed even after managing to sleep

The Mind-Body Link

The study of psychoneurophysiology examines the link between mind and body, and how the function of either can affect both elements.

Your mental thoughts, i.e. your internal dialogue, have the ability to influence every single cell in your body. How? This is via the hypothalamic-anterior pituitary-adrenal axis and how this communicates with the body via your sympathetic nervous system. As a chiropractor I primarily address a physical problem as most people present to me with physical pain. However, I clearly recognise the two-way link between physical and mental wellbeing. I know that physical stress and mental stress are linked and can be affected in either direction. So, just as negative internal dialogue may stimulate a negative stress response, so positive mental internal dialogue may stimulate a positive response. As you can see from the three main pyramids of Framework, Fuel and Feel, all of these contribute to overall Function. The Mind-Body link is crucial in this overall picture because stressors due to any of the factors discussed within Framework, Fuel and Feel will contribute to your overall 'environment'.

By improving someone's physical wellbeing, chiropractic adjustments have the ability to decrease cortisol (one of the major stress hormones) levels, reduce the effects of depression and also improve your immune function.

Ways to improve your mood

I will cover energy levels later, but are there any easy hints to help you, or a loved one, raise their mood? Yes!

- Spend time with friends: We know that one sign of feeling down can be to withdraw from socialising. But getting out, spending time with friends and having a laugh are all very important.

- Get a massage: Massage can play a fantastic role in relaxation and feeling better, so I like to educate that massage really can feel great and help you physically and mentally. Massage reduces cortisol levels and simultaneously raises serotonin. Serotonin is a neurotransmitter that has a very important role in raising mood, reducing anxiety and increasing happiness. Other powerful functions of serotonin include blood clotting and sexual function.

- Mood boosting foods: These are foods that are high in serotonin such as walnuts, kiwi fruit, bananas, tomatoes and plums.

- Omega-3 fish oils: The many benefits of these essential fatty acids have already been discussed. However, in this specific case we know that if your ratio of omega-6 to omega-3 is out of balance, it is likely to have a significant effect on mental health. In extreme cases it has been demonstrated that prisoners, sentenced for very violent behavior, exhibit a very large imbalance. Take omega-3's to boost how you feel.

- Play with a dog: Man's best friend can really help you here. Your fluffy canine friend cannot help but lift your mood and this is due to many factors, including that you are moving around and feel the love from your dog.

Focus also means mindfulness to me. This is one of my personal 'Achilles' Heels'. I am a 'doer' and find it hard to stop and stand still for a moment. There is always something else to do right now! However, both you and I need to commit even a little time to stop and unwind, to regain focus. Research has compared groups practicing various forms of mindfulness and looked at the effect it had on telomere length in the cells. A yoga group showed that they maintained their telomere length when compared to a comparable group of non-yoga people. Clearly, an activity such as yoga can, and will, benefit both the mind and the body.

E: Environmental

Environmental factors that can affect how you feel are many and I am not going to go into detail in some of these complex areas. Rather I do want to make you aware of these, as they will play a massive role in the health of anyone affected adversely.

All the factors within this section are stressors that affect us, or someone we know, from the outside in. Often the person struggling with issues feels trapped and helpless. If you do suffer from any of the issues below, you need to find help to speak about it, or look how to reframe the challenge that faces you. If you recognise any of these challenges affecting a friend, family member or loved one, then you may be the catalyst needed to help them work their way through. What is certain is that any of these challenges, whilst not easy to change, must be changed or they will eventually cause a significant reaction in mind or body or probably both.

Work, finance and housing

- Work/Life Balance: On the surface this may not sound too serious. However, an imbalance of work/life is extremely common and its effects can be insidious and incremental. I don't think many people who are in employment feel underworked too much of the time. What is that proverb? "All work and no play makes Jack a dull boy." We should all endeavour to find sports, hobbies and passions that we get excited about and that make all the hard work worthwhile. The mental and physical benefits of these are fantastic.

- Feeling unhappy at work: If you are working very hard, but are finding work either too hard or too boring, it can make you unhappy. Are you under-appreciated? Do you feel like a tiny, insignificant cog in a vast machine? Do you feel insecure in your employment? Do you work for yourself or have you taken the leap into entrepreneurship and are now responsible for a team and for their futures as well? Whilst some people thrive in high-pressure work environments, many people struggle on silently, fearful of their job security if they raise any concerns.

- Lack of Money: Both the previous two scenarios may be linked to this one. Money pressures are very common, and for people with many different levels of income. Anyone who starts to live beyond their means will feel a terrible burden from ongoing pressure.

- Housing: If you feel the pressure to maintain the roof over your head, I guarantee that there is a 100% probability of feeling stressed and anxious. This will also be the case if you are struggling to afford suitable quality housing, especially if you have children.

Relationships and upbringing

Many people have expectations put upon them, whether by their parents, partner or spouse, or through cultural expectations. If these expectations feel incongruent with the affected person, this can be a cause of great anxiety over a long period of time.

Society pressures

Some of the many pressures of modern life have already been discussed. However, it is worth reiterating that the demands upon most of us have changed radically in the last 50 years or so. The environment in which we live has evolved at a crazy pace. The cost of housing often means that both parents need to work, and work normally means very long hours. This pressure is pushed onto our children as well. School generations ago was all about learning, but now there is constant monitoring, and as parents are so busy children get to spend less time with them than ever before.

We get less sleep now, eat processed food and are exposed to ever-increasing levels of air pollution. The end result is increased stress on both our minds and bodies. This whirlwind lifestyle can lead to many things, but can certainly cause adrenal fatigue, due to overwhelm.

Levels of depression are constantly increasing, and suffering depression is now very common. There are many theories as to why this is the case. Many people live hectic lives and feel under pressure from work and paying the bills. There is now less time than ever to maintain social relationships (I don't mean on Facebook) with our friends, let alone in our local communities or within our own families. Healthy social interaction has been replaced by too much television, news media and other developing technology. If you suffer from depression, or love someone who is depressed, then you need to engage in more real social interaction, rather than less.

Whilst there are many societal pressures that may cause mental stress, I want to focus on a few areas, the pressures on women, children and those who suffer traumatic events.

Despite it being the year 2018, there are still many specific pressures on women of any age, compared to men. We see higher levels than ever before of teen suicide, depression and other mental health issues in teenagers, obesity levels continue to rise (even more so in young women than men) and teen pregnancy levels continue to rise.

Peer pressure is a constant problem, as it always has been. However, as access to and perceived importance of media, including social media, become more and more invasive, there seems little escape. Teens look at movie stars and photo-shopped models and feel uncertainty over their body shape. The temptation to experiment with alcohol and other drugs persists.

Are there solutions to this myriad of challenges? Yes, but before the solutions are in place we need to stop some of the problems! We see a massive decrease in physical activity and sport across all age groups. As the amount of sport has decreased at schools, what precedent does this set for that generation as they progress through the rest of their lives? We need to eat less processed foods, and ensure that we have enough good quality sleep, to allow rest and recuperation.

Traumatic events

Trauma will undoubtedly have a huge, and often sudden, effect upon health and wellbeing. This traumatic stress causes a sudden overload of negative stimulus, leaving you in shock. This may include bereavement, sexual or physical abuse, being on the receiving end of bullying and/or violence or the shock of a relationship breakdown.

I have worked with patients who have come to me for help from physical pain who have been suffering from such traumatic events. It became self evident that a woman recovering from the trauma of rape, or someone suffering the loss of a partner or equivalent, felt that they benefitted greatly from their chiropractic care. They felt that as well as relieving their physical symptoms, they 'felt lighter' and more relaxed as care continued, even if their symptoms had been present for a while.

E: Energy

Your mind is one of the biggest contributors to energy levels, both physical energy as well as mental energy. Having great levels of energy allows you to feel alive, be much more productive and happier! So how can you boost your mental energy levels?

1. Be Grateful: I am sure you have regularly heard the expression, "count your blessings", and yet this phrase flies over many people's heads. I realised some time ago that I have been guilty of this myself at times. In the hustle and bustle of our very busy everyday lives it is easy to think of the glass being half empty, rather than half full. You should take stock and remind yourself of what you have to be thankful for.

   ACTION: Get yourself a pen and paper. Write down a list of *at least* 10 things that you are grateful for.

2. Find Positive People: It was Jim Rohn who famously said that you become the average of the five people you spend the most time with. Have a look at the five people you spend most time with. Are these

people reflecting how you want to be, aspiring to life how you would like to? We are all social beings, but can shy away from social interaction if we are unhappy or depressed.

ACTION: Are any of your friends a negative influence on you? Decrease your time with any negative influences, and increase your time with the positive influencers. Who are your top five influencers? I know that some people get trapped in a cycle that makes them unhappy, but the first step is to recognise this and then you have to be brave to make some changes.

1. Be Positive, Think Positive! This may sound very simple, but for some it is a real challenge. You need a strategy to maintain consistency.

   ACTION: Start writing a journal. This may only take as little as 15-20 minutes every night. Writing a positive affirmation and what you have to be grateful for that day can make you realise why you should be feeling positive. Verbalising these positives makes them real.

2. Go Outside! Get up, leave the house or the office and get some sunshine. Increase your vitamin D levels and increase your energy levels. Sunshine also raises your mood quickly.

   ACTION: If you get tired at work, leave the desk and go outside. Develop this habit as you need to microbreak regularly, not just to improve your mental energy levels but also for all the benefits to your framework and musculo-skeletal health.

3. Have More Fun! Ensure that you plan ahead and make time for your family, partner, and friends. Likewise, prioritise activities and hobbies that you are passionate about. Remember that "All work and no play makes Jack a dull boy".

   ACTION: Plan ahead: Set times for activities and hobbies. Set a 90-day rule to escape for a mini-break with your nearest and dearest.

4. Declutter you mind: The aim here is to simplify things that you do every day. Simplification decreases stress, increases productivity and stops you wasting mental energy.

   ACTION: Set a timetable for yourself and plan ahead. Set reminders in advance. Delegate away unimportant tasks. Decrease your time spent on social media. Finally, and I think most importantly, DO NOT watch the News. The news media only ever brings you worry and stress, as it is their job to fill 24-hour news-streams with something worrying!

5. Try Meditation: Meditation and mindfulness can be extremely relaxing and can calm your mind brilliantly. I personally find stopping, even for a moment, a great challenge. However, you can find guided meditation that may take just a few minutes to do.

ACTION: Find a guided meditation that feels right for you. You may need to try several types, and you can find meditation apps now that can be downloaded easily on your smartphone.

6. Live in the present: This one is simple and powerful. Look forward, don't look backwards. It is too easy to fester in the past. Never live your life in regret of decisions made. Those decisions / actions / life events have happened. Accept that they have happened, and then move on looking forward. Never live in the past.

L: Love

"Where there is love there is life."

~ Mahatma Gandhi

Love yourself

I am too old, or I am too young. I am too fat, or I am too thin. I am not clever enough. I am not good looking. Ask a large group of people for their good points and bad points. The list of bad points will always overwhelm the length of the list of good points. We are very hard on ourselves but this affects our mental wellbeing. We need to be kinder to ourselves.

The study of somatoneurophysiology examines the relationship between our physical being, our mind and the human physiology. We understand that physical stress can send pain signals to the brain, affecting our mental health.

Likewise, negative mental thinking will have a negative effect on both the mind and our physical being.

So, a positive mental attitude will create good, healthy, proprioceptive messages that stimulate better physical function. A negative mental attitude creates increased levels of nociceptive (pain giving) signals to the body. Love yourself to feel better in both mind and body.

Loving someone with depression

Anyone suffering from depression tends to feel isolated and they withdraw from social interaction and contact. More and more people feel lonely with increasing numbers of people living on their own. I believe it was Mother Theresa who said, "The most terrible poverty is loneliness and the feeling of being unloved."

Depression can often make someone feel like a burden to those who love them. They need help, but usually are not seeking help and may be wary of accepting help. You will need to tell them, repeatedly, that you love them, unconditionally. Tell them why you love them, thereby reminding them of all their positive strengths, and do not mention any negatives. They are all too aware of their perceived negatives.

The mind-body link is very real. As well as getting your depressed loved one up and about, use some, or all, of the tips I recommended to improve mental energy.

ACTION: Sit up really tall for me. Lift your head and chin up to look at the ceiling. Open your eyes wide, and make the biggest smile you can! Hold this position for at least 15 seconds and keep that smile wide. I dare you to tell me that you did not feel great, or even a little manic!

Being a little bit manic is great for your soul. Your body produces serotonin and other natural 'happy' chemicals. Depressed people will respond in exactly the same way. So, find lots of opportunities for fun, laughter and silliness!

Being depressed usually occurs over a long period of time, and is not a flash in the pan. Depression usually runs along, hand-in-hand, with feeling fatigued. One of the very best medications for fatigue and depression is exercise. Try to get out and about to exercise for about 30 minutes every day. This does not require you to join a gym, put on legwarmers or wear a sweatband. It can be a simple brisk walk for 30 minutes or a couple of 15 minute walks. By inviting your loved one to go with you for a walk is a great way to try and increase their energy, decrease their depression and benefit from all the massive benefits of regular, moderate exercise.

Chiropractic effects on your mind and body

Chiropractic research demonstrates very good results for improving joint motion, increasing proprioceptive feedback to the brain, and decreasing painful nociceptive feedback. I have already stated that normal physical or mental health requires the body to be in balance, i.e. displaying homeostasis. By understanding how the two-way neural process works between the mind and the body, we can understand how the benefits of chiropractic (or osteopathic) care, regular moderate exercise and positive thinking can create very similar benefits to each other.

If that is the case, then we can also see how the negative effects of loss of normal spinal function, being too sedentary and negative thinking can all cause adverse effects to your mind and body.

These effects can be excited by physical adjustments, or by stimulating the brain and central nervous system, via neural stimulation.

I have written throughout this book about healthy proprioceptive (normal movement) signals to the brain and unhealthy nociceptive (abnormal or no movement) pain signals. Within every muscle of your body are receptors that are called muscle spindle fibres. These spindle fibres measure muscle movement and activity and constantly send these messages to the brain so that it can continuously construct an image of body position and function. The muscles that have by far the highest concentration of muscle spindle fibres are those found in the neck, just below the back of the skull. The density of these spindle fibres is so high that it has been judged that positional feedback (of the head and neck) to the brain is not their sole function. Instead this is the primary source of balance and proprioceptive feedback for the whole body.

Movement stimulates the brain with healthy, proprioceptive signals. If for example you have a restriction in normal spinal movement, then that area will send nociceptive (pain) signals instead. One of the side effects of this is the release of the stress hormone cortisol. Chiropractors call these areas of restriction 'subluxations'. Chiropractic adjustments can effectively remove the subluxations and restore normal proprioceptive signals to the brain from the previously restricted segment. Subluxated segments need not be painful either. The reduced function can cause loss of postural feedback to the brain even if there are no symptoms present.

As cortisol breaks down, some of its by-products are natural depressants that lower mood, and make you feel tired.

Chiropractic, in the purest form, is all about improving spinal motion and aiming to restore this action to normal. As the Nobel Prize winner, Dr Roger Sperry, said, "90% of the stimulation and nutrition to the brain is generated by the movement of the spine." That quote is in the window of my Spinal Health Centre! Spinal motion does not only concern spinal function. As Dr Sperry knew, spinal motion is necessary to ensure mental function which is itself 100% necessary as it controls ALL other functions in your body. Chiropractors and osteopaths are the leading experts in restoring spinal function. Correct spinal function is essential if you expect your physiology to be working as it should.

7

The Function Pyramid

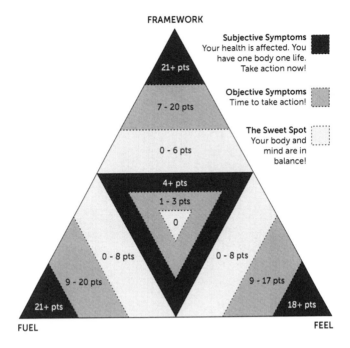

Figure 14: The Function Pyramid – One Body One Life

By now you I am sure you will realise how the three areas of Framework, Fuel and Feel are all equally essential to ensure healthy function.

For human function to be balanced is just the same as when I was in my rowing coaching days. A rower can be assessed by looking at their technique, physique and mentality. You will not find an elite rower who is weak in one of these areas; it is simply impossible. Likewise, it is impossible to have proper function if you are struggling in just one of the areas of Framework, Fuel or Feel. However, you cannot assess these areas in terms of obvious symptoms or signs of sub-optimal function in any of these pyramids.

As with our imaginary rower, we need to predict these areas of weakness and train ourselves to start doing what is required to pre-empt an issue in any area.

Ideal function lies within the centre of the Function Pyramid. If you are in the middle section, then you have areas to improve, your function is not ideal, but you may or may not be demonstrating any apparent symptoms of poor functional health. If you are in the outer zone of the pyramid, then there are obvious things that you should be addressing urgently to improve your function. If your function is in this zone, then your health is either at risk or is giving you clear and evident symptoms of dysfunction.

What is your overall function from each of the pyramids? Take this short quiz to give you an indication of where you currently sit. I have kept it as brief, yet effective, as possible to provide you with an accurate appraisal.

Where do you sit in the overall Functional One Body One Life Pyramid?

If you are in the normal zone of each of the Framework, Fuel and Feel Pyramids, you score zero points towards your function score.

Being in the middle zone of every pyramid scores 1 point. While symptoms may not be obvious, sinister or worrying you yet, they are indicative of abnormal function and change is needed!

Being at the peak of each pyramid is indicative of significant subjective symptoms, with urgent change needed, and scores 3 points.

What score determines your position in the pyramid?

0 points   To be in the healthy centre of the pyramid you may not be perfect, but you will be in the normal zone of each of the three pyramids that create function.

1-3 points   Any points ensure you will be in the middle zone at least. However, you can be here if you are in the severe zone of one area and normal in the other two.

4+ points   You need to take action urgently as your functional health is poor and your health is significantly compromised.

8

The One Body
One Life Quiz

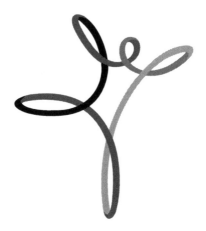

Framework Quiz:

1. Averaging over a week, for how many hours per day do you sit still? (include work time, commuting and at home)

   a. Less than 6 hours per day
      0 pts

   b. Between 6-12 hours per day
      1 pt

   c. More than 12 hours per day
      3 pts

2. Do you exercise (i.e. brisk walking or more) for at least 30 mins every day?

   a. Yes
      0 pts

   b. No
      3 pts

3. How do you breathe?

   a. Does your chest rise and fall?
      3 pts

   b. Do both your chest rise and belly expand?
      1 pt

   c. Do you belly breathe only?
      0 pts

4. Test your balance: NOTE – Please be careful here if you are not confident with your balance. Test this near something to grab onto, such as a door frame or the back of a sofa, or have someone with you. Perform this test barefoot, and repeat on each side three times to take an average result. Can you balance for:

    a. Less than 20 seconds with your eyes open?
        3 pts

    b. More than 20 seconds with eyes open?
        1 pt

    c. More than 20 seconds with eyes closed?
        0 pts

5. Stand barefooted. Look straight ahead and feel balanced. In this position and without changing your posture, can you:

    a. Raise your toes without changing your balance?
        0 pts

    b. NOT raise toes without changing posture?
        3 pts

6. Do you suffer from back, neck or joint pain?

    a. No, no pain anywhere
        0 pts

b. Yes, mild aches and pains
1 pt

c. Yes, regular back, neck or joint pain
3 pts

d. Yes, and I have had back surgery, a history of 'slipped disc', or suffer from Sciatica
5 pts

7. Do you suffer from headaches, including migraine?

a. No, I never get headaches
0 pts

b. Yes, occasional mild headaches
1 pt

c. Yes, I get regular or severe headaches
3 pts

8. Have you ever had your foot and ankle biomechanics assessed, and if necessary foot orthotics prescribed?

a. No, I have never had this checked
1 pt

b. Yes, and all was fine, no action needed
0 pts

c. Yes, and I have had orthotics prescribed
0 pts

d. Yes, I have been checked, I need orthotics but I have not ordered these yet
3 pts

9. Do you perform core strengthening exercises, to improve functional core and spinal stability and mobility (this may include Pilates and/or yoga exercises)?

a. Never
3 pts

b. 1-2 times per week
1 pt

c. 3 times or more per week
0 pts

10. Do you visit a chiropractor or osteopath at least once per month to maintain, and improve, your Framework function?

a. Yes
0 pts

b. No
3 pts

Your Results:

0 – 6 pts   You are within the normal zone.

7 – 20 pts   You are in the middle zone. Things to improve but you may not have many obvious signs of symptoms.

Over 21 pts   You are in the danger zone. Almost certainly you have clear symptoms of loss of normal function in your Framework. Take action now!

Fuel Quiz:

1. How hydrated are you? Be honest now! Google 'urine colour chart for hydration' and you should find a standard urine colour chart. A standard one will have 8 colour levels. A golden rule is: levels 1-3 is normal wee, 4-8 and you need to hydrate!

   a. Level 1-3 (hydrated)
      0 pts

   b. Level 4-6 (dehydrated)
      1 pt

   c. Level 7-8 (severely dehydrated)
      3 pts

2. Do you supplement your diet with high quality omega-3 fish oils?

   a. Yes
      0 pts

   b. No
      3 pts

3. Do you supplement your diet with probiotics or eat natural fermented foods (i.e. kefir, kimchi, sauerkraut) at least 3 times per week?

   a. Yes
      0 pts

   b. No
      3 pts

4. Do you smoke?

    a. Yes
        0 pts

    b. No
        5 pts

5. How many portions of fruit and vegetables do you eat per day?

    a. Less than 5 per day
        3 pts

    b. Between 5-10 per day
        1 pt

    c. More than 10 per day
        0 pts

6. Do you base your main meals around starchy foods, e.g. potato, rice, pasta or bread?

    a. Yes
        3 pts

    b. No
        0 pts

7. Regarding foods that contain sugar. On an average day how many portions of these foods do you eat or drink? (one portion will equate to: one glass of fizzy

drink, two biscuits/cookies, one bowl of breakfast cereal, spoon of sugar in tea/coffee, a small chocolate bar, sweets or slice of cake)

    a.   None
           0 pts

    b.   1-2
           1 pt

    c.   More than 2
           3 pts

8. Do you drink LESS than 2-3 units of alcohol a day if you are a woman or 4-5 per day if you are a man?

    a.   Yes
           1 pt

    b.   No
           3 pts

    c.   I am teetotal
           0 pts

9. Regarding your exposure to pollution:

    a.   Do you live in the centre of a large town or city? Y/N

    b.   Do you work in the centre of a large town or city? Y/N

    c.   Is your home or workplace adjacent to a busy road? Y/N

   i. Zero Ys
       0 pts

   ii. One Y
       1 pt

   iii. 2-3 Ys
        3 pts

10. If you are feeling hungry between meals, what is usually the first thing you reach for?

   d. Nothing or water
       0 pts

   e. A piece of fruit or vegetable
       0 pts

   f. A biscuit or snack bar
       3 pts

Your Results:

0 – 8 pts   You are within the normal zone.

9 – 20 pts   You are in the middle zone. Things to improve but you may not have many obvious signs of symptoms.

Over 21 pts   You are in the danger zone. Almost certainly you have clear symptoms of loss of normal function to the Fuel your body is running on! Take action now!

Feel Quiz

All these questions should relate to the last TWO weeks.

1. How often have you had little interest in, or pleasure in doing things?

   a. Not at all
      0 pts

   b. Several days
      1 pt

   c. More than half the time
      2 pts

   d. Nearly every day
      3 pts

2. How often have you been feeling down, depressed or helpless?

   a. Not at all
      0 pts

   b. Several days
      1 pt

   c. More than half the time
      2 pts

   d. Nearly every day
      3 pts

3. How often have you found yourself struggling to fall asleep or stay asleep?

    a. Not at all
        0 pts

    b. Several days
        1 pt

    c. More than half the time
        2 pts

    d. Nearly every day
        3 pts

4. How often have you been bothered by a poor appetite or by overeating?

    a. Not at all
        0 pts

    b. Several days
        1 pt

    c. More than half the time
        2 pts

    d. Nearly every day
        3 pts

5. How often have you been bothered by feeling fatigued, very tired or been suffering from low energy levels?

    a. Not at all
        0 pts

    b. Several days
        1 pt

    c. More than half the time
        2 pts

    d. Nearly every day
        3 pts

6. How often have you caught yourself feeling bad about yourself, feeling like a failure or like you have let your family down?

    a. Not at all
        0 pts

    b. Several days
        1 pt

    c. More than half the time
        2 pts

    d. Nearly every day
        3 pts

7. Have you had an anxiety or panic attack?

    a. Yes
       3 pts

    b. No
       0 pts

8. How often have you felt nervous, anxious or very worried about something?

    a. Not at all
       0 pts

    b. Several days
       1 pt

    c. More than half the time
       2 pts

    d. Nearly every day
       3 pts

9. How often have you found yourself being quick to anger, easily offended or too irritable?

    a. Not at all
       0 pts

    b. Several days
       1 pt

    c.   More than half the time
         2 pts

    d.   Nearly every day
         3 pts

10. Have you been worrying about any of the following things?

    a.   Your health
         Y/N

    b.   Your weight
         Y/N

    c.   A strained personal relationship
         Y/N

    d.   Stressed about your work
         Y/N

    e.   Financial worries
         Y/N

    f.   Struggling about a bereavement
         Y/N

    g.   Stressed about your family
         Y/N

    h.   You've nobody to turn to for help
         Y/N

    i.   Little or no sexual desire
       Y/N

        i.   If zero Ys
           0 pts

        ii.   1-2 Ys
           1 pt

        iii.   3-4 Ys
           2 pts

        iv.   more than 5 Ys
           5 pts

Your Results:

0 – 8 pts   You are within the normal zone.

9 – 17 pts   You are in the middle zone. Things to improve but you may not have many obvious signs of symptoms.

Over 18 pts   You are in the danger zone. Almost certainly you have clear symptoms of loss of normal function due to the Feelings your body is suffering! Take action now!

9

The One Body
One Life Blueprint

Whilst I would never say that every twist and turn in our health can be controlled, I do believe that following the Feeling Alive Blueprint will create a predictable pathway to improving your health, and maximising your health potential.

The problem most people face is that they do not know where to start, take action sporadically, fall back into bad habits, or simply do not realise why taking action is so important for their health.

The Feeling Alive Blueprint follows the Feeling Alive Pyramid and breaks down into 10 sections.

Framework

1. **S**tructure and spinal dysfunction

2. **P**oor posture

3. **I**nnate breathing

4. **N**eurological integration

5. **E**xercise and physical conditioning

Fuel

6. **H**ydrate for life

    Eat well

7. **A**bsorb

    Life supplements

Feel

8. Focus

9. Environment

Energy

10. Love

Step 1...

Structure and spinal dysfunction

The Number 1 priority is to be pain free. It is impossible to start improving your overall health and wellbeing if you are struggling with ongoing pain. I recommend chiropractic or osteopathic care, NOT only to relieve your pain, but to ensure that your spinal function is restored as much as possible.

Step 2...

Poor posture

As your pain is being relieved then your posture needs to be normalised and maximised. You want to ensure that your posture is balanced, healthy and in balance. Posture is not just about appearance, but is 100% necessary for optimal human function. You need a posture expert who will rehabilitate you, and teach you how to continue to work on your posture at home.

Step 3...

Innate breathing

You must remember how to breathe correctly. As babies we all take deep, easy, breaths. As we age, the combination of poor posture and chronic stress causes us to take very shallow breaths with our chest; we start to pant. You need to be taught how to breathe again, and then to maintain this during postural and functional exercises.

Step 4...

Neurological integration

After physical and postural stress have been reduced it is essential to ensure that your neural function is balanced and congruent. This can be achieved by specific Neurological Integration, balance training and therapeutic massage.

Step 5...

Exercise and physical conditioning

This is a very important section to ensure improvement to your overall function. The aim of the exercise and physical conditioning component of the Health DNA Blueprint is not to transform you into a gym god or goddess. Instead, it is to ensure that you are fit enough, functional enough and strong enough to maintain normal function, form and posture during your activities in daily life. This section is varied depending on the specific individual but comprises regular brisk walking (treadmill walking is fine), spinal rehabilitation exercises and core strengthening, and therapeutic massage.

Specific advice for those aiming for certain sports or sporting targets would be set for that individual.

Step 6...

Hydrate for life and eat well

Hydrate your body properly and consistently. Calculate your body weight in pounds (lbs) and divide by 2. This tells you the amount of fluid ounces you need to drink. Make this easier to understand by converting to what you know. Multiply by 0.0625 to tell you the quantity in pints. Multiply by .0296 to calculate in litres. If you drink a mug of caffeinated coffee, or alcohol, you need to add a similar amount of water to your normal daily intake.

Eat like our ancestors evolved to and attempt to avoid processed food and refined sugar. Primal Eating takes us back to the basics and natural food. Don't panic as this can still be super yummy! At this stage let me make this really simple. In an ***ideal world*** the ideal primal eating pattern would mean:

- No processed foods

- No sugar and other refined carbohydrates

- No grains

- No dairy

- No alcohol

- Eat like a wolf, not like a podgy bear – i.e. do not overeat!

- Avoid like the plague – high fructose corn syrup, trans fats, monosodium glutamate, aspartame

- Eat lots of fresh vegetables – raw, steamed or lightly cooked

- Fish, meat – grass-fed meat

You should also minimise refined sugars and trans fats from your diet as there is nothing beneficial in these. High sugar levels will massively raise your risk of developing diabetes, and possibly increase your cancer risk. Trans fats are man-made, and raise the risk of Type 2 diabetes and cardiovascular disease.

Step 7...

Absorb and life supplements

Much of what you absorb is genuinely tricky for many people to control, and I completely understand this. For example, it is tricky to not work in the polluted air of Central London if that is where your home or work is. However, if you smoke then you should stop! If you cover yourself with lots of make-up, and other body lotions and potions, look to reduce this. Be cautious with the sun, but ensure that you, and your children, get at least 20 minutes of sunshine on your skin, every day.

Life Supplements include several essential sources of nutritional support. Whether for yourself or a child, we should all ensure that we add high-quality omega-3 fish oils, Vitamin D, probiotic foods (whether from natural fermented or supplemental sources), magnesium and antioxidants.

Step 8…

Focus

The ability to focus, and identify, one's thoughts, to maintain attention and recognise one's mood. The study of psychoneurophysiology examines the link between mind and body, and how the function of either can affect both elements. As part of the programme at my Spinal Health Centre, we utilise BrainTap technology as well as therapeutic massage to relax, reduce stress and reset.

Step 9…

Environment and energy

Work/life balance, feeling unhappy at work or a lack of money can all contribute to adversely affecting your personal environment. All these types of stress are likely to have an adverse effect. Anyone suffering from these ongoing anxieties and worries will also suffer from reduced energy and a feeling of fatigue and lowered mood. I recommend meditation and mindfulness exercises as well as a combination of exercises to combat these. I also utilise BrainTap technology, and guided meditation, to challenge many of these issues very efficiently.

Step 10...

Love

Be kind to yourself, and feel confident in your own skin. Somatoneurophysiology examines the relationship between our physical being, our mind and the human physiology.

A positive mental attitude will create good, healthy, proprioceptive messages that stimulate better physical function. A negative mental attitude creates increased levels of nociceptive (pain giving) signals to the body. Love yourself to feel better in both mind and body. I recommend exercises and again the BrainTap technology to stimulate effective change.

About the Author

Andrew Green is a passionate, honest and informed communicator. He has developed his bold communication style whilst working in the diverse roles of chiropractor and rowing coach. Andrew was selected as part of the medical team for the London 2012 Olympic Games and also works with Premiership and Championship football teams. Always open to new thinking and passionate about sharing ideas, he is an authentic and empowering educator and coach. Having completed his Master's in Chiropractic in 1999, he also holds the International Certified Chiropractic Sports Practitioner qualification.

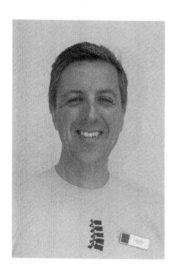

Printed in Great Britain
by Amazon

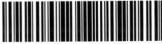

45512883R00120